HEALERS

HEALERS

Extraordinary Clinicians at Work

David Schenck
and
Larry R. Churchill

OXFORD
UNIVERSITY PRESS

OXFORD
UNIVERSITY PRESS

Oxford University Press, Inc., publishes works that further Oxford University's
objective of excellence in research, scholarship, and education.

Oxford   New York
Auckland   Cape Town   Dar es Salaam   Hong Kong   Karachi
Kuala Lumpur   Madrid   Melbourne   Mexico City   Nairobi
New Delhi   Shanghai   Taipei   Toronto

With offices in
Argentina   Austria   Brazil   Chile   Czech Republic   France   Greece
Guatemala   Hungary   Italy   Japan   Poland   Portugal   Singapore
South Korea   Switzerland   Thailand   Turkey   Ukraine   Vietnam

Copyright © 2012 by Oxford University Press, Inc.

Published by Oxford University Press, Inc.
198 Madison Avenue, New York, New York 10016

Oxford is a registered trademark of Oxford University Press

Library of Congress Cataloging-in-Publication Data

Schenck, David.
Healers : extraordinary clinicians at work / by David Schenck and Larry R. Churchill.
p. cm.
Includes bibliographical references.
ISBN 978-0-19-973538-9 (hardcover)
1. Alternative medicine. 2. Physician and patient. 3. Healing.
I. Churchill, Larry R., 1945- II. Title.
R733.S328 2011
610—dc22

2010041077

9 8 7 6 5 4

Printed in the United States of America
on acid-free paper

David Schenck dedicates this book to
Judith, Carol, and Ed,
who taught me that healing was possible.

Larry Churchill dedicates this book, with deep
gratitude, to
Roy, Tobi, and Keith,
masters of the healing arts.

David Schenck and Larry Churchill together
offer special thanks to
the 50 clinicians whose wisdom we have sought to
reflect in this volume.

CONTENTS

CONTENTS

ACKNOWLEDGMENTS

The authors would like to thank those who made the composition and completion of this book possible.

For contributions to the manuscript:

John Mulder, M.D., for his willingness to let us use an unusually large portion of our interview with him as the anchor for Chapter 3, "How Healing Happens: Reports from the Field," and for his willingness to be identified as the source of this critical material.

Tessa Carr, Ph.D., for making available to us her doctoral dissertation, "Recovering Women: Autobiographical Performances of Illness Experience," for Chapter 5, "Patient Perspectives: Healing from the Other Side of the Bed Rail." Discussions with her of early drafts of this chapter were instrumental in bringing it into its published form.

Mark Smith-Soto for permission to use his marvelous poem "Intensive Care" in Chapter 5.

Eve Henry, M.D., who as a Vanderbilt medical student did an extensive study of the placebo effect and the psychoneuroimmunology of healing and wellness, and subsequently became our coauthor for Chapter 6, "The Biology of Healing: Neuroscience and the Education of Healers."

There were two other significant contributions to Chapter 6. David P. McCallie, Jr., M.D., gave the chapter a thorough and insightful review. His generosity has resulted in a far stronger chapter. Elizabeth Claydon and Michael Putnam, while undergraduates at Vanderbilt, provided imaginative research assistance in the areas of psychoneuroimmunology and placebos that proved valuable for the eventual shape of the chapter.

Scott Neely for his careful review of Chapter 8, "Ethics and Medicine: Healing the Wounds of Fate," and his as ever trenchant editorial recommendations.

For assistance in the production process:

Our dedicated transcriptionists, Denise Lillard, Cathy Mann, and Malinda Mabry-Scott, for the care with which they handled this essential task.

Two editors par excellence, whose timely assistance was invaluable: Katie Haywood for her marvelous job of reformatting and organizing the materials in preparation for publication, and Allison Adams, for her keen eye, good sense, and relentless attention to commas.

At Oxford University Press, Editor Peter Ohlin, Assistant Editor Lucy Randall, Production Editor Susan Lee, and Project Manager Smitha Raj have been uniformly helpful and supportive.

We were also fortunate to have as a reader for Oxford University Press Professor Kathryn Montgomery. We thank her for her immediate recognition of the aims of the book and enthusiasm for it, and for the suggestions that made the final product stronger than it would have been otherwise.

For institutional support:

From the beginning of this project we have received financial support from the Baptist Healing Trust of Nashville, Tennessee. We are most grateful to the officers and the Board for their confidence in us, and for believing that a study such as this would bear fruit. We want to especially thank the former President and CEO, Erie Chapman; the current President and CEO, Cathy Self; and the Director for Educational Programs at the Trust, Kristen Dinger.

We are also grateful to the Eben Alexander Fund at Vanderbilt for early and ongoing financial assistance.

Both of us are nested in a community of scholars, researchers, clinicians, and teachers within the Center for Biomedical Ethics and Society in the Vanderbilt University Medical Center. This has been a most commodious environment for both the germination and the writing of this book. We thank our colleagues, past and present, for their support, and especially the Center's Director, Dr. Ellen Wright Clayton.

David Schenck would like to thank:

Charlie Reynolds for launching a career of inquiry—into ethics, practice, and medicine—whose circuitousness neither of us anticipated.

Glenn Graber for guiding my first observations of clinicians at work.

John Wood for dozens of peripatetic conversations about ethnography, interviewing, and the understanding of culture.

Jonathan Imber for 30 years of intellectual friendship. Our discussions of medicine, modernity, epidemiology, and character have shaped my thinking on nearly every topic covered in this book.

My teachers at Joseph's House—Blossom and Cathy, Patty and Priscilla, and all the residents—for showing me how presence, respect, and compassion can heal.

Dee and Mac Rhodes, my sister and brother-in-law, for inviting me into their home, giving me a place to work and to live, for 2 months during the time this manuscript was written. Likewise, my sister and brother-in-law Patti and Harry Cocciolo, for providing their summer home for 2 months for me to continue with the book. One could hardly ask for more generosity and support than these four offered.

Finally, my mother, Dolly McGinn, for her early support of this research, and her continued enthusiasm for it.

Sande Churchill, who has sponsored my professional life and nurtured my intellectual life for nearly 40 years, beginning when I was an undergraduate studying ethics and religion at the University of North Carolina–Chapel Hill. The life of the mind I have lived and loved would never have unfolded as it has without her friendship.

And, finally, a word or two about the delight, the edification, the ongoing sense of accomplishment that has been my day-by-day, month-by-month, year-by-year experience of working with Larry on this volume, as colleague, as coauthor, as friend. Not to mention his diligence and creativity in finding institutional and financial resources to support our projects as they have progressed. No one could imagine, much less ask for, a better partner in any such work.

Larry Churchill would like to thank:

My wife, Sande, for the web of love and support she has provided over more than four decades. This volume is different and better than it would have been without her, in ways perhaps only she and I will recognize.

My coauthor, David, for his generosity of spirit in collaboration, his clarity of insight at critical junctures in the writing, and his ongoing friendship.

INTRODUCTION

A physician, working abroad in a makeshift clinic for indigent patients, sees that his next patient has no legs and is being carried into the office by his family. The physician instinctively begins to imagine how he can help this man. He likely needs prostheses and crutches, maybe extensive diagnostic procedures and further treatment for whatever medical condition caused the loss of his legs. "We couldn't get him into a chair, so the nurse and I both decided to sit with him on the floor. We got down and met him eye to eye and asked, 'How are you?'" Here the physician was readying himself to hear a litany of medical problems resulting from the absence of legs. "My eyes are going bad," the patient said. "I make shoes and can't support my family with failing eyes." The physician was astonished: "We go to the eye clinic. We find him some glasses, and he goes back to work." Against all expectations, a patient troubled by his eyes—not his lack of legs—was helped almost immediately and was enormously grateful. "This patient thought we were God himself," the doctor said.

This is a book about healers and healing. We begin with this small encounter of the patient with no legs to highlight the idea that healing can take many forms, some anticipated and some not—as in the example above—and some involving mundane conversations while others involve dramatic interventions. Healing, whether ordinary or extraordinary, and sometimes both, always has to do with the quality of relationships. It always has to do with connections between people that make us whole and restore us to the deep sources of meaning for our lives. Just as this cobbler with no legs was restored to his fundamental role as provider for his seven children.

Healing is frequently discussed but seldom studied in a systematic way. When we are patients seeking care or clients seeking help we recognize that the quality of the relationship can be beneficial to us. Trust and confidence in those who are seeking to help us can have profound healing effects. Most of us choose to continue to see our doctor, nurse practitioner, therapist, acupuncturist, or other health-care professional because the relationship "works," because these helpers would be willing to get on the floor with us and engage us eye to eye. Thoughtful professionals also recognize this relational factor at work in the healing of their patients, and some are legendary for their ability to make a difference in the health or well-being of those they assist.

Regrettably, these relational skills are under the radar in many professional training programs. Frequently the assumption is that when it comes to relational skills, "you either have it, or you don't," with the implicit message, "If you don't, we can't teach it to you." Obviously this assumption becomes a self-fulfilling prophesy and a tacit endorsement for neglecting everything that can't be easily measured or reimbursed as a technical skill. Physicians, for example, are compensated large sums for their skill in passing a lighted tube down the throat or slicing open the abdomen, but nothing for reassuring patients prior to these procedures or interpreting the results to them afterward. The great scientific prowess in health care we have achieved over the past century has made many practitioners quite robust technically, but underdeveloped relationally. This has profound implications both for those who seek help and those who endeavor to provide it.

Obviously little progress can be made in this area unless we seek greater understanding of how healing works, and what skills are essential for becoming a healer. Leaving healing relationships to the province of luck or inborn abilities means that we will continue to neglect them educationally and that progress here will be grudgingly slow. The irony is that what is evident to us when we are in need of help is hardly acknowledged when we are well and designing curricula, or assigning monetary value to professional skills.

If we are ever to do a better job of educating professionals to be healers we will have to understand the dynamic of healing relationships, what makes them work, what makes them fail, why some helping professionals learn to become healers and why others never rise above the level of technical competence. This book is a report on what we have learned in our effort to study healers and healing skills in a more systematic way.

Both of us have spent our lives in health care. Churchill has been educating medical students, hospital house staff, nurses, and chaplains in academic medical centers since 1973. Schenck has worked in a wide range of nonprofit healthcare organizations: as an administrator, as a community organizer for health services, and as a chaplain in hospital and hospice settings. Both of us have seen firsthand how the relational dimension of professional help is sometimes the difference between good and bad outcomes. Even when outcomes are unfavorable, finding meaning in the problems is powerfully affected by the ability to elicit trust and to empathize with others, as well as by commitments like shared responsibility, loyalty, and deep respect for the humanity of another person. This book is an effort to put on display what we have learned from interviews with 50 clinicians recognized by their peers as healers, lessons that we believe speak not only to doctors but to the broad spectrum of professionals who work in health care.

We have both been deeply humbled by what we have learned, and by the responsiveness of the people we interviewed. We learned much about healing, but we also learned what a rare and valuable thing it is to be able to discuss healing, to be able to reflect on powers that both seem beyond us and yet reside in us as human beings. A short version of our research findings was reported in 2008 in *Annals of Internal Medicine*. Many of the numerous responses we received from physician readers were remarkable and gratifying, but none more so than that of an Italian physician who wrote that reading the article was a healing experience for him, confirming the part of his work he found most meaningful.

We hope clinical educators reading this book will pay more attention to the phenomenon of healing, and will be motivated to improve both their skills and those of their learners. We hope the general public will feel that some of the things they most prize in professional helpers are beginning to be recognized and valued, and will demand greater competence in these skills from those who make claims to help them.

* * *

We begin in Chapter 1 with a report of interviews with 50 clinicians over a 2-year period, clinicians identified by their peers as expert healers. Their responses to the questions we posed were sometimes obvious and remarkably simple, at other times surprising and complex. They consistently engaged the subject of healing by offering practical advice—describing things they do, rather than discussing ideas or concepts. The audiotapes of these interviews comprise over 600 pages of transcripts. Our analysis of this material clustered around eight themes, each described as a practical skill. We have sought to remain true to the form of the responses, and have couched these skills as imperatives— things to *do* with patients and clients, rather than ways to think about them. Mastering these skills would provide enduring improvements for patients, just as practicing these skills consistently would provide the most enduring rewards of patient care for clinicians.

Many of the practitioners we interviewed recognized that patient care inevitably involves ritual processes. Chapter 2 steps back from a focus on healing skills as separate capacities to consider how they function together as elements in a larger ritual structure. In Chapter 3 we turn our interpretive lens to a finer focus, this time explicating and interpreting one particularly fruitful interview in detail.

Caring for the sick has always been of extraordinary importance to human beings and, coupled as it now is with the power of modern science, parallels and interconnections between healing in health care and healing in religious and spiritual traditions are natural and inevitable. These parallels and interconnections are the subject of Chapter 4.

But what about the patient perspective on healing? In Chapter 5 we review some of the most articulate and prominent patient narratives about illness and clinician–patient relationships, from "the other side of the bed rail."

One of the most exciting facets of healing is the amount of recent research on the biological pathways involved and the subsequent rethinking of just how healing occurs. Chapter 6 reviews the considerable amount that is known from scientific studies on healing, drawing from work in behavioral science, physiology, neurology, immunology, and placebo studies. In this chapter we argue for a rethinking of the placebo effect as an element in a larger phenomenon we term the "healing response." Here we also make suggestions for a model of medical education that would integrate training in healing skills more completely into health professions curricula.

All of our informants recognized that their power to help others is closely intertwined with their own well-being. Healers need wholeness in themselves to evoke the healing potential inherent in others. One of our interview questions sought to elicit ways that professionals sustain their health and find wholeness in the midst of very demanding practices. This is the focus of Chapter 7.

In the final chapter we connect healing with ethics, focusing on an ancient but largely neglected understanding of ethics as a healing art. Modern understandings of ethics assume it is all about making sound decisions. But ethics also involves traits of character, before and after choices and decision points; ethics is often a matter of how one's life is shaped by the routines and rituals of daily work. These interconnections are often lost in our fixation on decisions, but the link is apparent in some of the earliest schools of Western moral philosophy. It is this connection between healing and ethics that we examine in Chapter 8.

Perhaps all authors have a sense of the right way to read their works, or at least a hope that readers will come with a set of assumptions that are commensurate with the authors' intentions. We are no different. Readers familiar with our previous works might expect the common topics and arguments of bioethics. This is not a bioethics book, at least not in any usual sense, nor does it feature ethical reasoning in the typical way. Our major purposes here are expository and interpretative. We are trying to be true to what clinicians have told us, to put on display and develop the threads that are evident from a special set of conversations with practitioners. At each turn we have tried to follow where the interviews led us, rather than make a theoretical case out of our findings. In some chapters we have provided a modeling of our findings, either on standard biomedical grounds, or in terms of humanistic and social science paradigms. But this has all been in the service of exploring our data, rather than the usual efforts to prove or disprove a thesis. Our hope is that the reader will read the entire book, and especially the tables, charts, and boxes, not as definitive conclusions but as pedagogical devices to assist in moving our understanding forward.

We do not advocate in this volume for any specific philosophies or schools of healing, such as conventional medicine, vitamin therapy, spiritual healing, or alternative and complementary approaches. A literature search on "healing" brings up books on religious or spiritual healing through practices such as prayer; on healing through alternative therapies such as diet, megavitamin therapies, and chiropractic and massage techniques; on healing mediated by pets, music, sex, and a variety of other means. Our aim is not to promote any one method or modality, but simply to describe in detail what actions are known by our clinicians to work in bringing about healing in people who are sick or in need.

We are convinced that the capacity to develop healing relationships is largely a skill set that can be taught and learned, and that professional education in the 21st century will need to incorporate what is known about healing relationships, just as the 20th century incorporated knowledge from the biological, social, and behavioral sciences. In the future the public will demand professionals who have relational competence as well as scientific competence. If this book can further that agenda we will have achieved one of our main goals.

HEALERS

[1]

HEALING IN HEALTH CARE: EIGHT THINGS THE BEST CLINICIANS DO

We thought we could cure everything, but it turns out we can only cure a small amount of human suffering. The rest of it needs to be healed.

—Rachel Naomi Remen

At the center of medical ethics is the healing relationship.

—Edmund D. Pellegrino

Physicians and patients alike recognize that their relationships can have healing effects. Compassionate, trusting relations between patients and practitioners are the chief delivery vehicle for the scientific interventions of modern medicine. Clinicians are concerned on a daily basis with convincing people to undergo physical examinations, accept probes into their private lives, endure diagnostic tests, take medications, or agree to surgeries that are inconvenient, painful, and sometimes hazardous. Relational skills are fundamental to success in these persuasive endeavors, and relationships themselves have potential therapeutic value—described in scientific terms as the "placebo effect"[1] or the "meaning response,"[2] as well as in ethical terms, as Edmund Pellegrino notes.[3] In addition, relationships with patients are a large part of the intrinsic rewards of medical practice.

Despite the general recognition of the importance of physician–patient relationships, the skills necessary for practitioners to establish and maintain healing interactions with patients are rarely studied systematically,[4] and are often consigned to the unscientific and mystified "art" of medicine and health care. The result is that education in this area is typically sporadic and *ad hoc*. Students and residents complete their training with widely varying degrees of competence in building relationships with patients. Some are superbly equipped to relate to their patients and clients. Some are so inept that they drive patients away and occasionally harm them inadvertently through their lack of attention, compassion, and care.

The study described in this book was motivated by the conviction that relational skills in patient care are not mystical attributes, but practices that can be identified and taught. While there are numerous volumes on interviewing,[5] and studies of physician–patient conversations,[6] there are few empirical studies of how physicians build relationships that have healing potential.

FINDING OUR INFORMANTS ON HEALING

During 2006–7 we interviewed 50 practitioners using a semistructured approach. The clinicians we recruited were regarded by their professional peers as especially good at establishing and sustaining excellent patient relationships. To identify our informants we asked: "Who among your professional peers possesses great skills in relating to their patients?" When a name came up repeatedly we knew we had found a person we wanted to interview. Our sample was drawn from university-based and community practitioners, and from urban and rural practices. We interviewed practitioners from three states in the southeastern United States, and included practitioners across a wide range of specialties: internal medicine, surgery, psychiatry, urology, pediatrics, dermatology, anesthesiology, family practice, and palliative medicine. In addition to M.D.'s, we also interviewed 10 practitioners from complementary and alternative medicine (CAM), similarly identified by their peers as having exceptional talents in healing interactions with their patients. Participating CAM practitioners also came from a variety of disciplines: chiropractic, traditional

Chinese medicine, massage therapy, craniosacral therapy, and midwifery. The age range of interviewees was mid-30s to late 70s, with equal participation from men and women.

We interviewed practitioners face to face, usually in the practitioners' offices or adjacent conference rooms. Whatever relational skills these clinicians possessed, we thought, would be more evident in person, and might not be conveyed through telephone interviews or written responses. Surveys conducted through questionnaires would have yielded a far larger sample but less depth of information. Although costly in terms of time, our interviews permitted a degree of detail and follow-up that otherwise would not have been possible. Most interviews took an hour or more. Although three participants we hoped to recruit did not respond to our initial letter of invitation, no one declined participation after learning more about the study. This was itself a remarkable endorsement of the need for greater understanding of the phenomenon of healing. Most participants welcomed what they termed a "rare opportunity" to talk about an important but neglected aspect of their practice. Interviews were audio-recorded, and the transcripts of the interviews were anonymized. We conducted the first 10 interviews and coded the transcripts from these first 10 together to establish a consistent way of interpreting what we were hearing and establishing our categories of interpretation. We then worked independently in interviewing, with both of us reading all transcripts, and reconciled any differences in interpretation for the remaining 40 transcripts. Our study was approved by the Institutional Review Board, a committee charged to review the scientific quality and to protect research participants, at Vanderbilt University Medical Center.

WHAT 50 EXTRAORDINARY CLINICIANS TAUGHT US

This chapter focuses on responses to the first questions of the interviews: *How do you go about establishing and maintaining healing*

Table 1.1 HEALING RELATIONSHIPS INTERVIEW GUIDE

---

1. How do you go about establishing and developing relationships with your patients? What concrete things do you do to bring this about?
2. In your experience, when and how does healing occur? Is healing something you try explicitly to do—or is it something that just seems to happen along the way?
3. Have you had experiences as a patient that have taught you important things about healing or relationships in health care?
4. What activities that promote wellness, wholeness, and healing do you personally engage in?

---

relationships with your patients? What concrete things do you do to bring this about? This was the first of four clusters of questions we asked. Table 1.1 shows the list of questions and the order in which we proceeded. We discuss responses to the other three sets of questions in later chapters of the book.

A note on the presentation: we use numbered, headings to express the major themes we encountered. Bulleted imperatives underneath these headings summarize the advice we heard about specific actions and attitudes. The eight major themes and specific suggestions listed below are all presented in the imperative mode. This is consonant with how the information came to us. Expertise in establishing and sustaining therapeutic relationships, our practitioners insisted, is not theoretical knowledge, but various kinds of "know-how"— action-oriented, goal-directed understanding. The message we heard again and again was couched as practical advice, essentially: "Do this."

1. Do the little things

- Introduce yourself and everyone on the team
- Greet everybody in the room
- Shake hands

- Smile
- Sit down
- Make eye contact (as appropriate)
- Give your undivided attention
- Be human, be personable

Though it may seem odd that the complex interactions between practitioners and patients that result in healing should begin with what used to be called the "common courtesies," the virtually unanimous testimony of our extraordinary practitioners is that the "little things" are key. The little things turn out to be big.

> One of the things that I routinely do is when I enter the patient's room . . . I try to make a point, of course, to make eye contact and to shake the patient's hand. I will often acknowledge anyone else that they have in the room with them, their significant others. So there are just certain obvious social gestures that are common in any new relationships that I try to establish right away.

Especially important is acknowledging all people in the room, including family members and significant others, and everyone on the medicine team. A small community is being formed, very quickly and under unusual circumstances. The practitioner has enormous power to set the tone and direction for this little community in the first encounter.

> I try to always look the people in the eye. I try to listen mostly [on the] first visit, and I take notes. . . . I think it shows them that I want to get it right. Patients are more likely to trust me if . . . I work to try to understand what they want me to know foremost.

Small gestures and actions, like note-taking, may speak far more effectively to a patient's need for trust and safety than repeating reassuring phrases.

If someone feels connected, then you're miles ahead in terms of being able to effect some sort of positive result and impact on the patient. So it's really establishing a positive, unique relationship where the patient remembers you. *Touch* is an extremely important part of that—so walking in, shaking hands, hand on the shoulder. Those sorts of things are very, very important.

One of the things I do . . . particularly when I see people in my office, or when I'm working in the clinic, I never have anything between me and the patient. . . . I've always had my desk up against the wall, and I just turn around and leave my stuff on the desk, out of the picture, because I'm not doing anything but talking with the patient.

In his book *Blink*, Malcolm Gladwell points out that as a species we seem to be hardwired to size up people and situations with amazing rapidity.[7] Perhaps this is one of those traits that have an adaptive survival function, for example, in sensing danger or safety with great rapidity and then forming an appropriate response. The expert healers we interviewed were saying something similar. Judgments about practitioners are often made quickly, if not literally in a blink, in a very short time. Encounters with patients, especially the initial one, must be marked by a kind of reassuring engagement, an offer of availability, safety, and a helping relationship. Once this happens, when the connection with the patient is established and the small community formed, there is a much better chance that the wide range of the practitioner's knowledge and skill then can be brought into play.

2. Take time

- Be still
- Be quiet
- Be interested
- Be present

Important as first impressions may be, however, beginnings that are courteous may show themselves to have been mere formalities unless these initial openings are followed by genuine presence. Presence requires a slowing down that lasts long enough for the practitioner and the patient to move past first impressions—and first anxieties. Patients typically wonder, "Will the doctor listen to me?" or "When will I get interrupted?" It is the practitioner's willingness to be still and be quiet that demonstrates that there is space.

> So my first meeting, though, is to try to get acquainted, and what I know is that it takes time, and for me to be in a hurry—I may have a thousand things going, but I need to go and sit down and try to look relaxed. I might even take off my coat, and try to give them body language that [says], "I have time for you."

Taking time makes it possible to listen with care to the answers generated by practitioners' questions.

> I start teaching in the first encounter, but I spend a lot of time listening to the answers to the questions that I ask, and then I try to let some silence take place, especially in people who are very concerned, so that they can tell me what they're concerned about.

Taking time is also important for the practitioner. Again and again those we interviewed said that it is the power of the human encounter in response to illness that keeps them going.

> I'm always eager to see a patient. They're all so interesting; every one of them, really.

Taking time is a way of honoring the other person and building the relationship, of showing that it matters. Taking time is a basic way of giving another person attention, and a precondition for a relationship. But time here is not primarily "clock time," measuring in minutes, although some minutes are obviously required. Rather, time for healing is measured in qualitative units. This can be illustrated in terms of two Greek words. *Chronos* is quantitative time, clock time—time measured uniformly in minutes, hours, and days. *Chairos*, by contrast, refers to qualitative measures of time: when something happens at the "right time," or "time that is full" regardless of its length, what sometimes goes under the contemporary cliché "quality time." Times in which one is "still, quiet, interested, and present" are chairos, and it is this understanding of time that healers have mastered. Readers may still think that this sort of qualitative investment in patients will require more quantitative units, more minutes, with patients, and of course sometimes this is true. Still, Platt and Gaspar claim that "a skilled physician can obtain a useful sketch of a patient as a person in less than a minute," and studies consistently show that permitting patients to state all their concerns, and not just their presenting illnesses, does not add substantially to the length of interviews.[8]

3. Be open and listen

- Be human
- Be vulnerable
- Be brave
- Face the pain
- Look for the unspoken

Why are being open and listening important? Because patients bring not just their ailments, complaints, injuries, and anxieties to physicians, but their whole, wounded selves, what Pellegrino called their "damaged humanity."[9] Only a small percentage of the hurts, pains, and anxieties people experience rise to enough significance to occasion a doctor's appointment. For most of us, by the time we make a visit to a practitioner we have tried and failed to solve the problem with our own resources, and/or we are sufficiently worried about ourselves that when we reach the practitioner's office the help we need is not just physical, but some combination of social/psychological/ spiritual. If we brought ourselves in to be fixed in the same way we deliver our cars to be repaired, there would be no need for openness and attentive listening.

There was constant emphasis in our interviews about the ways in which helping others means being open to their humanity—seeing "them" as persons like "us"—and this implies an awareness of one's self that is more than professional. Hence, "be human" and "be vulnerable" are grouped with this constellation of imperatives, and the command to be brave or courageous naturally follows. It takes courage on the part of the practitioner to be willing to open up to, and be opened by, the woundedness of patients over and over again. And yet our informants claim that it is just such willingness and courage that makes healing possible.

> You have to be honest. You might be able to help a lot of times—it depends, but listen to his story. . . . You listen for the wound and you let them know that you have wounds. You are not perfect.

Part of why this makes healing possible is that when the practitioner models such willingness and courage, the patient has permission to follow suit and offer the same. And here immense power is generated.

> You know, I might get tearful, or I might get upset, and so I think a lot of physicians, at that point, pull back, become more clinical, and move through it, but if you stretch a little bit, and you allow yourself to feel those emotions, it helps the patient tremendously. It actually is very rewarding, as much as it's difficult.

Being open, and being willing to be vulnerable, both begin with deceptive simplicity—they begin with listening:

> Listen, listen, listen, listen: that's my mantra inside my head. Shut your mouth and listen. Let these people tell you what they need to tell you.

A study of Beckman and Frankel showed that among 74 office visits, the mean time a patient was allowed to talk before being interrupted by the practitioner was 18 seconds.[10] Not all patients were cut short in their opening statement, but most were, and of those who were interrupted, only one was afforded the opportunity to complete his or her opening statement. Of course what occurs after an interruption can be a meaningful dialogue, and dialogue can be a vehicle for identifying and coming to know the patient as more than a collection of symptoms. Alternatively, interruptions can be driven by the desire for greater efficiency in the interaction and a desire to more quickly and precisely locate the medical problem. This is, of course, very important to do, but our informants were clear that such a laser focus, especially early in a patient conversation, forecloses the potential for the interaction itself to carry healing potential and sometimes leads to inferior care. We will return later to the ways that failure to listen can jeopardize patient well-being.

An important part of listening is listening for stories, for the narratives that give coherence to the lives of one's patients.

Any opportunity . . . to listen a little bit to their life story; I found out early on that being able to listen to their life story connected me better with that child and that family, and then we had a relationship.

The teller of the story shares his world by recreating it for the listener—and the listener becomes co-creator of that world by receiving the story, and often reinterpreting key parts of it.[11]

Listening is the most important thing, I believe. Asking about them, not just about their disease. Letting them tell their own story without too many interruptions. Caring about the aspects of that story.

There seems to be a natural human hunger for telling one's stories and for one's story being heard. Novelist Reynolds Price says that the need for such telling and hearing is as deep as the need for food, shelter, safety, or sex. His book *A Whole New Life*, which describes the new person who Price became following treatment for a spinal cancer, is vivid testimony to his thesis.[12] We live by stories, by the stories we tell ourselves, by how others of importance receive these tales and interpret them for us, and by how we learn to re-narrate them, incorporating their changes, shifts, and surprises. Visits to professional helpers are in a deep sense the offering up of a story that needs an interpreter: "I am worried I have a cancer. Can you help me find out if I do and help me to deal with it?" This encapsulates one kind of story that gets presented to practitioners—but never, of course, in the first 18 seconds, or in this matter-of-fact declarative way. We do not "report out" but "narrate," a far more intricate and interesting act. Doctors and other professional helpers are recipients and interpreters of some of the major narrations of our lives. Healers know what a privilege this is and have learned to listen, as they said to us, "with the third ear," "for what is unsaid." And for the deeper currents evident in the tears, the hand gestures, the shifts in body posture that indicate when the narrative is at an important turn. Jerome Bruner calls these turns "what knocks the story line off expectancy."[13] One healing skill is, then, learning to hear, and—as the clinician said above—"caring about the aspects of that story," that particular unique tale that discloses just that person and no other.

But sometimes listening becomes very difficult. Sometimes stories are horror stories, soaked in pain and fear, and here again skill in hearing is central, since the fear may be unwelcome or threatening to face. An intensivist we interviewed put it this way:

> Fear comes out as anger. Families don't want to come in and express they're afraid that their loved one is going to die, and often, it will masquerade as anger. And I need to be prepared for however this is going to come out, and I need to not run from it.

We do not usually think of listening requiring vulnerability, risk, and courage. But often it does, and just as often it becomes a gateway to healing.

4. Find something to like, to love

- Take the risk
- Stretch yourself and your world
- Think of your family

Seeking in every patient a quality, an achievement, even just a mannerism that can be appreciated or admired mobilizes a particular capacity in caregivers. Jerome Groopman, in his book *How Doctors Think*, has underscored the importance of finding something to like about one's patients.[14] He describes an instance in his residency training in which a patient's complaints "sounded to me like a nail scratching a blackboard" and how he became deaf to what this patient was saying about her illness. The patient died a few weeks later from an aortic rupture, which Groopman says he had failed to diagnose because he had fixed on another interpretation of her symptoms. He concludes, "Physicians who dislike their patients regularly cut them off during the recitation of symptoms and fix on a convenient diagnosis and treatment . . . developing a psychological commitment to it." He continues, "Strong negative feelings about the patient make it harder . . . to abandon that conclusion and reframe the clinical picture differently."

Groopman believes some degree of compassion, some emotional investment in patients, is protection against misdiagnoses. Our informants put forward a similar thesis about healing more generally, saying compassion is critical, as both a precondition for healing and an element of healing, to both the patient and the practitioner. This was a strong theme from our interviews. Compassion, it should be noted, does not entail emotional entanglement when properly engaged, but should be seen as an investment of positive caring energy in the patient.

For certain practitioners, such an investment is a foundation of their practice:

> What I tried to do when someone came to my office is to not only take a very full and complete history, but to show the patient that I was very willing to become involved in his life. . . . My way

of practicing for my entire practice life was to bond very closely with my patients, and to start that bonding process at the first meeting.

But this involvement cannot, of course, come only from rote behaviors or gimmicks—it must be based in something real:

I took a class with a famous psychiatrist who taught techniques of patient conversation—including recommendations to "lean forward" and to "sit on the front edge of your chair." I asked, "Wouldn't it be better to just be interested in your patients?"

For some practitioners it is useful to imagine the patient as being like their parents or their spouse or their children or grandchildren, depending on the age and gender of the patient. Once the caregiver feels empathy and opens to compassion, another whole realm can open up:

I have a heart and soul which I can offer them, which is the way of bringing them some love. Love is a tough word to talk about when you are talking about doctor and patient relationships. Do you love your patients? I think you have to. Some people don't want to say that they do, but I think in order to really get to the point of healing you have to love. You have to be compassionate, understanding, and willing to walk the wounded path with them.

"Love" here is not so much an emotion as a quality of heart and soul—and it manifests itself most authentically and most powerfully in compassion and understanding. To find these capacities in themselves, practitioners have to be "willing to walk the wounded path" with their patients.

We're in it for the moment where there's that double heart open connection of love and truth. . . . It makes my practice doable.

5. Remove barriers

- Practice humility
- Pay attention to power and its differentials
- Create bridges
- Be safe and make welcoming spaces

Once inside the healing space, our best practitioners said they seek to remove as many barriers to a genuine person-to-person encounter as possible. Barriers can be of many sorts. Some are physical; some are attitudes. Removing barriers often involves an appreciation of the power differentials between doctor and patient, and the way these differentials can be lessened by humility.

> I'm not too good to open a door or roll a patient back into a room. And I'm not too proud to wipe the snot off a crying mother, or empty a trash basket . . . [or] to do any of those things that the lowest-ranked employee of the hospital does.

Another clinician put it this way:

> I like to have them understand that I am a human being, that I am not a god. I am a physician.

Humility is a virtue in many religious traditions. While these theological understandings clearly influenced some of our informant practitioners, their greater emphasis was on a more basic under-standing that is reflected in the etymology of "humility," rooted in the Latin *humus*—earth. The meeting ground for practitioner and patient should be the common ground of recognizing the basic humanity, the *humus*, from which we all come and to which we shall all return. Removing barriers, whether physical or attitudinal, is important precisely because barriers hide this common ground on which clinicians and their patients or clients can meet. Sometimes the common ground is "on the floor," as in the story of "the patient with no legs." Common barriers are desks, computer screens, white coats, or assumptions about whose time is more important. In brief, humility is one essential ingredient in the move to establish connections on a human and not just a medical basis. This allows the range of the provider's nonprofessional life and interests to come into the relationship in a natural way. Here's one example:

> I just have an interest in a lot of different things. We have season tickets to the symphony and season tickets [for the football team], and we'll just have this mixture, involvement in the arts, and volunteering here in [local city], and I try to do all of these different things, and it really—it comes in very handy when you're trying to communicate with all different types of people.

6. Let the patient explain

- Listen for what and how they understand
- Listen for the fear
- Listen for the anger
- Listen for expectations
- Listen for their hopes

Earlier we talked about the fact that patients are storytellers, and the importance of getting to know patients' stories—the narration of who they are and what is important in their lives. We now focus more specifically on *explanations*—that is, on that portion of patients' stories that constitute their current complaint. For example, practitioners commonly ask, "What brings you to the office today?" and this is usually posed even after a reason has been elicited from the receptionist and physical signs, such as blood pressure, temperature, and so on, have been gathered by the admitting nurse. Now we are focused on the patient's understand of *why* he or she has come.

Our informants insisted that patients are often the best source of information on their condition, and in this sense an explanation of *why* is a history that should never be ignored. But in addition, our informants said that just hearing patients' reasons for seeking help, even if it yields nothing in addition to what can be discerned though diagnostic tests, can be an essential part of healing. Patients need not only to be heard, but to know that they are being heard, so creating an environment in which the patient's explanation has a natural place is essential. For these reasons, open-ended questions seem particularly effective.

A good way to get the patient started is just asking them what they understand about what's going on so far. And that's a very broad opening; it allows them to either be very scientific and talk about the tests that they've had . . ., or it's an opening if the emotional piece is important to them at that time.

Immediately the practitioner gets an understanding of what the patient will be able to hear and hence be able to understand.

[This way] what they understand about what's going on can come through right at the beginning: "What I understand is that I'm in a lot of pain, and I'm very scared, because X, Y, Z." So it gives them an opportunity to frame it for what they need the most, rather than immediately starting with specific questions about the medical side.

Then the practitioner can begin a process of education and guidance, using language the patient is comfortable with or requires. As the patient talks, the caregiver looks for the opening, the place to insert a comment or an insight—the place to go to further the healing process.

One clinician described the sequence in which this occurs in her practice:

First there's making comfortable and dropping my judgment, and second, there's listening, and then third is waiting for the cues, to see where is the invitation? . . . I'm talking to somebody, and you know when they're ready to hear something. You know, when I am listening, there is just a knowing of when the words can come, and so I wait for the opening, and I learned that in school, too, because we talked about being the needle.

Notice the way in which these components build on each other: establishing a place of comfort and safety, dropping judgmental postures and demeanors, inviting an explanation and waiting for an appropriate opening, looking for a place to enter effectively, as if inserting a needle. While this might sound like an excessive degree of passivity by the practitioner, in fact listening and waiting attentively are very active. They are active but not aggressive. They are intended to enact a commitment to nonviolent communication, actively inviting explanation, seeking it early in the interaction and on the patient's terms, rather than forcing the conversation into professional categories. We are not, of course, suggesting that every patient encounter can or should have this character; this is clearly not a demeanor for the emergency or operating room. But in the office, and especially as relationships are being established, this actively engaged, often-silent reception of the patient's explanation can have powerful effects.

7. Share authority

- Offer guidance
- Get permission to take the lead
- Support patients' efforts to heal themselves
- Be confident

Many practitioners establish their expectation of shared responsibility for healing at the very beginning:

One of the initial parts of my consultation with somebody is that I'll tell them today's visit is all about ascertaining whether I can help you or not. "I'll make some recommendations to you. [But] you will always dictate what you want to do."

For this shared responsibility to become shared authority—a rather more difficult relationship to establish—the practitioner must view the patient as a "fellow expert":

> What's often not recognized is the patient brings a particular level of expertise, too. Who knows more about them than them? And after all, it is about them, and how they are able to get better.

For the patient to be a full partner, however, the practitioner must have a confidence that projects itself into the relationship. Patients must trust the practitioner's ability to hold the healing space securely, and to provide guidance as they move together down the "wounded path":

> And so I think a lot of it, for them, is a sense of perceived confidence, and that has to do with the way you interact, the way you speak about options, the confidence you that have in your own skills.

A cardiologist put it even more starkly:

> Lack of confidence by the doctor has doomed many a therapy. The first step in really healing the patient is to be confident.

In Chapter 6 we will talk about the way in which confidence and the expectation of being helped can have marked effects on patients in terms of physiological responses to medications, or to comforting touch or verbal encouragement. For now we are simply outlining and illustrating the major themes from our interviews. It is apparent that whether or not practitioners were aware of the studies we will discuss—and most were not—they had a deep intuitive grasp of how being confident in the face of patient complaints, worries, and anxieties elicited beneficial patient responses.

It might be thought that confidence would be contradictory in light of what we have reported earlier about the virtue of humility.

However, confidence does not mean cocksureness, or assertions of infallibility or guarantees of help, any of which would indeed be inconsistent with humility. Confidence is most often a "quiet confidence," not loud proclamations, which ironically serve to raise doubts about the abilities or judgment of the practitioner. Confidence, as seen on the faces and felt in the hands and words of clinicians, seems to provide hope to patients who may otherwise be harboring anxieties and doubts. Some of our informants thought this element was so important that they schooled their staff and their teams to reflect the message to patients: "You are in a competent place where people know their stuff. We are willing and *able* to help you."

8. Be committed and trustworthy

- Do not abandon
- Invest in trust
- Be faithful
- Be thankful

Gestures of commitment and fidelity to a patient can be very simple and direct. One practitioner indicated he always finds a way to say this: "We are going to work this through together." A pulmonologist, often treating people with chronic, complex illnesses, had this expression of fidelity as a standard for his practice: "I may send you to see a specialist, but you will always come back to see me afterward." This is clearly a way of saying, "I will not abandon you or send you off with the idea of transferring your care"—what is known in medical jargon as "turfing," shifting the patient and his or her problems to someone else.

An addiction specialist put the loyalty motif even more forcefully, in advice that could have easily fit into several of the other seven themes, and expresses a demeanor of loyalty for dealing with the inevitable setbacks and failures that occur when patients do not participate in their own recovery: "Patients need to know that you love them even if they fail to adhere to treatments."

Patients may fear being abandoned, not only if they fail to adhere to treatments, but after improving as they consider leaving the relational environment that has facilitated healing. Hence, an intention and a plan to carry the healing power of the encounter out into the larger world are usually needed.

> One thing I always, always try to do is make sure that every patient leaves with a plan. . . . I will tell patients [this] is one thing you can always count on. You always leave with a plan with me.

But the plan, whatever it is, rests on a grasp of the patient's story. And here we come full circle. Being able to speak to that story is a chief ingredient in sustaining trustworthiness, and this contributes to good outcomes.

> Healing is about connections, and connections are about listening to people's stories. Listening to people's stories is what makes us trustworthy—and as we are found trustworthy we are able to be more effective.

The patient's story continues outside the consulting room or hospital. And the practitioner shows his or her recognition of and involvement in that story by promising not to abandon the patient as the story progresses.

> Your patients have to trust you. They have to trust that you have their best interests at hand and there's nothing that solidifies that trust like saying I value you as an individual. I value who you are, what you do, and what you contribute to my life. And because of that you can explicitly trust me and what I recommend to you.

Note the phrase "what you contribute to my life." One of the most consistent themes of our interviews was that finding meaning in medical practice is fundamentally connected to the capacity for forming patient relationships of real trust, and that such relationships are one of the principal rewards of doctoring. Readers surprised to find a bullet point under "Be committed" that includes thankfulness or gratitude will now see the logic to which we were made privy in the minds of our expert healers. The gratitude arises from recognition of the extraordinary privilege of being part of a healing process, and from having their own lives changed by these activities.

SUMMARY

Our findings are summarized in Table 1.2.

Our findings have several limitations. While we did reach saturation in terms of repeating patterns with 50 interviewees, it is always possible that additional interviews could have revealed additional healing skills, as might a different mix of practitioner specialties. Additionally, there may be differences between what clinicians say

Table 1.2 SUMMARY OF PRACTITIONER SKILLS PROMOTING HEALING RELATIONSHIPS

1. **Do the little things**
   - Introduce yourself and everyone on the team
   - Greet everybody in the room
   - Shake hands; smile; sit down; make eye contact
   - Give your undivided attention
   - Be human, be personable

2. **Take time**
   - Be still
   - Be quiet
   - Be interested
   - Be present

(Contiued)

Table 1.2 CONTINUED

3. **Be open and listen**
   - Be vulnerable
   - Be brave
   - Face the pain
   - Look for the unspoken

4. **Find something to like, to love**
   - Take the risk
   - Stretch yourself and your world
   - Think of your family

5. **Remove barriers**
   - Practice humility
   - Pay attention to power and its differentials
   - Create bridges
   - Be safe and make welcoming spaces

6. **Let the patient explain**
   - Listen for what and how they understand
   - Listen for the fear and for the anger
   - Listen for expectations and for hopes

7. **Share authority**
   - Offer guidance
   - Get permission to take the lead
   - Support patients' efforts to heal themselves
   - Be confident

8. **Be committed and trustworthy**
   - Do not abandon
   - Invest in trust
   - Be faithful
   - Be thankful

they do and what they actually do in patient encounters, discrepancies that might be identified through videotaping. Still, our work seems to pass one important test: a review of what patients have said in print largely confirms our findings. Chapter 5 is devoted to a review of some of the best-known examples of what patients have said about their illnesses, their clinicians, and their overall care. This review confirms that our practitioner interviews offer a reliable, if partial, portrait of relational healing skills.

In the quotations that open this chapter, Remen reminds us that healing skills remain central, while Pellegrino affirms that these skills are not just interactional strategies, but essential elements of health-care ethics. We will return to the connections between healing skills and ethics in Chapter 8. The benefits of mastering these skills repay the effort many times over, both in terms of improved patient care and in terms of the ability of physicians to find deeper meaning and fulfillment in their practices.

In the next few chapters we will unpack the elements of healing relationships. In Chapter 2 we examine what can be learned by thinking of how the eight skills discussed here work together as medical rituals, and in Chapter 3 we will trace the responses of one of our extraordinary clinicians more closely to see the fine detail of healing work.

[2]

MEDICAL RITUALS: ORGANIZING
THE HEALING ELEMENTS

While conducting our interviews of extraordinary practitioners, we began to recognize a recurrent pattern in their descriptions of the formation of practitioner/patient relationships. We want in this chapter to step back from the taxonomy of skills developed in Chapter 1 and examine the structure of this formation process. In so doing we will also revisit each of the eight core skills in that taxonomy, this time focusing on its contribution to that set of essential activities we now call "building the container."[1] We will use the metaphor of the container as a way to signal the delineation of boundaries and the necessary protection for what can be fragile and complex relationships. Our intention is to offer our practitioners' pragmatic perspective on those clinician behaviors that help to establish and sustain that container. We will argue that this dynamic in many ways mirrors archaic rites of passage.

Despite the widespread dominance of the biomedical model in industrial and post-industrial societies, there has remained recognition of the critical and legitimate role of religious ritual as an element of healing for vast numbers of patients.[2] On the other hand, there has been very little recognition within the culture of biomedicine, or in American culture at large, that medicine itself has from the beginnings of human society always been associated with ritual practices. Yet analytical study of the relationship of ritual, religion, and medicine has been going strong since the very beginnings of sociology and anthropology in the late 19th century. And now, with the ascendancy of medical anthropology over the past two decades, a renewed wave of studies describing the rites and rituals of medicine has emerged. These new studies are important in their own right but perhaps even more so in the part they may play in countering the stereotype of biomedicine as a field birthed in biochemical laboratories just after World War II, and developed through the decades since, as simply a series of evidence-based practices.[3]

References to rites of passage, and the foundational texts for their study by Arnold van Gennep and Victor Turner, are by now quite common in this recent literature on ritual and medicine. And we, too, have found ample evidence of the (mostly unreflective) practice of such rites in contemporary medicine. Our aim, though, is not add to the anthropological literature, but instead take one "operational step" past studying and describing medical rites of passage and show specifically how our practitioners understand their part, and perform their roles, in executing these rites.

THE RITUAL STRUCTURE OF HEALING SKILLS

Important ritual practices, anthropologists tell us, typically take the following form:

- Transition from ordinary life into a non-ordinary or sacred "container"
- Special activities and healing experiences within such a "container"
- Structured exit from the healing "container" back into the ordinary world

Using this framework, think of the average visit to a healthcare practitioner. One enters the office, fills out forms, talks with the practitioner's assistants, giving over one's health history and other normally secret personal information—this being the transition from the ordinary world into the non-ordinary world of the practitioner's office. Then follows a variety of activities not encountered, condoned, or allowed in the ordinary world. These activities, furthermore, are often ones that touch upon the most important aspects of self:

- Intimate conversation on major crises, wounds, illnesses, and suffering
- Intimate physical contact of various kinds
- Direct physical intervention in the body, including cutting skin, giving injections, inserting objects into a variety of orifices, probing deep tissue, adjusting spines, and sticking needles into sensitive areas all over the body

These activities are allowed in the privileged healthcare container because they induce certain experiences, either immediately or in the future, that are desired by the patient and by society. Such experiences may be described as ones of "healing": of pain being relieved, of return to important roles in society and the family, or of restoration of "wholeness," in a variety of physical, social, emotional, and spiritual senses. Finally there are rituals of exit—putting clothes back on, having bandages placed on exposed places, getting a prescription, making a plan of care for the patient to follow after leaving the office, setting an appointment for a next visit, paying one's money or offering insurance information, and walking out the door.

One way, then, to describe the skills of our outstanding practitioners is to speak of them as (1) skills that facilitate patient movement from the ordinary world into the specialized space of health care; (2) skills that deepen and hold that space where the healing work with patients is done; and (3) skills that facilitate the patient's exit from that out-of-the-ordinary space.

Reviewing the eight core skills identified in Chapter 1,[4] we would argue that the first two—*Do the little things* and *Take time*—are critical for the patient to make a successful transition through the liminal space separating the ordinary world from the extra-ordinary world of health care. The "little things" provide a non-threatening stepping-off point into the feared, and often dangerous, contained space where one focuses on illness and health.

ENTERING the CONTAINER

1. Do the little things
- Introduce yourself and everyone on the team
- Greet everybody in the room
- Shake hands; smile; sit down; make eye contact
- Give your undivided attention
- Be human, be personable

2. Take time
- Be still
- Be quiet
- Be interested
- Be present

WITHIN the CONTAINER

3. Be open and listen
- Be vulnerable
- Be brave
- Face the pain
- Look for the unspoken

4. Find something to like, to love
- Take the risk
- Stretch yourself and your world
- Think of your family

5. Remove barriers
- Practice humility
- Pay attention to power and its differentials
- Create bridges
- Be safe and make welcoming spaces

6. Let the patient explain
- Listen for what and how they understand
- Listen for the fear and for the anger
- Listen for expectations and for hopes

Medical Rites of Passage

EXITING the CONTAINER

7. Share authority
- Offer guidance
- Get permission to take the lead
- Support patients' efforts to heal themselves
- Be confident

8. Be committed and trustworthy
- Do not abandon
- Invest in trust
- Be faithful
- Be thankful

Figure 2.1

So starting off with trying to get in a position that doesn't make the patient vulnerable, and if you're in a setting like the emergency department, trying to ensure privacy and some quiet. And then making physical contact as well as eye contact. Usually, laying hands on the patient somewhere, when you first meet them and greet them, whether it's shaking a hand, or if they're too ill for that, a hand on the shoulder, something like that, to make a physical connection right at the first interface. And certainly, if there's family around, which there often is in such situations, making sure you know who the people are, and greeting them individually, before we start launching into the medical details.

It is often not only the patient who is making this transition, but the patient's family as well. For these patients to make the passage successfully, their families must make it, too. Correspondingly, there's a group of people on the practitioner's side who are a critical part of these transitions. One doctor puts it this way:

> Any doctor who cares about patients needs to have an office staff which can talk with patients which will be part of the therapy team. I don't care if you call that front office person a secretary, an office manager, and a billing clerk—I don't care, they're part of the treatment team.

An especially important role these staff members have is that of supervising the "geography" of the transition from the outer world into the medical world. These are the people who establish the tenor of the physical, emotional, psychological, and spiritual spaces that mediate between outside and inside. Though not examined carefully enough or often enough, the role of "the treatment team" in the healing process is critical. Even so, it is quite understandable that caregivers who work daily in these domains, and live constantly with their often tragic realities, often neglect the importance of the small things that ordinary people—that is, "patients" and "families"—need to get into their specialized world. Likewise, for practitioners and those who assist them, the transition into the world of the healthcare system can take place quite quickly, if not instantly. And thus it can be easy for them to forget that patients, and patients' bodies in particular, need time to make transitions well and fully, so that they can be fully and completely present once the engagement with their illness begins.

The next four of the eight core skills—*Be open and listen, Find something to like, Remove barriers,* and *Let the patient explain*—are the ones decisive for deepening the practitioner–patient encounter within the healthcare "container," and for strengthening the container itself. The patient has now crossed the threshold. Will the experience with the practitioner encountered within the container be profound or superficial? Will it be part of a full healing process, or will it be a perfunctory effort to manage one or two of the patient's symptoms? All this depends on how much trust can be developed between the patient and caregiver.

When I enter the patient's room, I make eye contact and shake the patient's hand, and I acknowledge anyone else that they have in the room with them. I introduce myself usually as "_____," and not as "Dr. _____." I then usually sit down with the patient and take a history, which is an unusual thing to do in dermatology. There is a tendency in private practice to do the physical exam first, or concurrently with the history, because the clues on the skin are so important. But I feel that patients aren't really ready for that— jumping right into the physical exam and baring themselves.

Here there is recognition that even when the patient is in the exam room, there are still degrees of deepening intimacy, and corresponding degrees of trust to be built. It is not that the history can't be done with the physical exam. It is, rather, that the overall relationship of the practitioner and the patient will develop more fully if these small moves towards more encompassing trust can be taken. And that trust, as we have seen again and again, is perhaps the most important and most powerful element in relationships that foster healing.

> So I will ease into it by at least taking a brief history. Another thing I do is always wash my hands in front of the patient, rather than just using that alcohol goop that is outside every room. I imagine the patient thinking, "That's a good thing. She's washing her hands before examining me." I usually do that after the history, while the patient is moving onto the examining table. So those are some of the rituals I do at the beginning of the encounter with the patient.

Note the use of the word "ritual." Some practitioners have a keen awareness of just what they and their patients are doing as these passages are negotiated.

On the practitioner's side, then, it is the ability to listen and be present, to find something in the patient to engage with positively, and to overcome barriers of class, gender, and race as effectively as possible. And that, in turn, makes room for the patient to offer more, to be more present himself or herself.

> Trust is developed when you're honest with people about what you're gonna do. You tell what you're gonna do. You give them the opportunity to participate any way they want to. "Do you want to put the speculum in yourself? Would that make you feel more comfortable? Or do you want to take this home and just try putting it in yourself, and then you'll know what it's going to feel like when I put one in next month?" Again, dealing with fear: "If you put your arm down like this, and we put the tourniquet on it, and bend it backwards . . . and look how it sticks up. We won't have any trouble. And I use the tiniest needles you can get, so it's not going to be as painful as you think."

These are the kinds of easily overlooked intermediate steps that are required if the patient and practitioner are to trust one another enough to move safely into more and more vulnerable material—and on to more and deeper encounters with the patient's woundedness, the caregiver's woundedness, and indeed the woundedness that marks the human condition.

And how do our practitioners speak of their role while the patient is within the container? The terminology, and the sense of responsibility, often have an archaic echo. One clinician says, "You are on a journey, and I can be your guide. I'll go down this path with you, but it is your journey." And another, "You've got to meet the expectations of the patient. You need to take the patient where they need to go medically and emotionally."

The imagery of the journey is ancient and archetypal, as is that of the guide. And as in the ancient stories, what we most want when we travel to the darkest and most terrifying places in life is someone who can say to us: "We have been here before. We know what to expect."

If I do enough of my own work and have experience going to my dark places, my scary places, then I know that it can be done. I know that it's healing. And so I'm not scared to take someone else there. I know it might feel uncomfortable and be distressing at first—but also incredibly healing. And so I will say, "We can go there. I'm not afraid. Do you want to go there?"

One part of having a guide—whether that guide was a shaman in a hunter-gatherer tribe, or a surgeon in the operating room of a major medical center—is having someone who knows the territory, who has been there before, who knows what you should be afraid of and what you really need not fear.

Another part of having a guide is having someone who will question you, reflect you back to yourself, challenge your assumptions and your sense of your own limitations. The guide thus functions at times as a mentor:

I try to hold up a mirror, and I know my colleagues do, too. Without judgment, holding up a mirror. Without shame, without blaming.

Just asking in one way or another, "Is this really what you want for your life in the deepest way, or is there another way? Is there another way for you to get what you really want?" Helping people find that, through dialogue, and just being present with them in a loving way and asking, "What is it you really want? Because your life is expressing in this way, and it's not getting where you want."

There is the invitation to move past one's perceptions of one's limitations, an invitation into a new life, and support for answering that invitation by beginning a new life based on an experience of healing.

There is, finally, one more blessing of having a guide that is just as important as the first two. And that is having the guide as a companion on the journey.

It's hard to go to those hard places alone. And so having a guide to mentor, to reinforce, to support going to really hard places is essential. I feel like I'm one of those people in modern times who take people where they need to go—where they kind of want to go, but are really afraid to go, but that will set them free. I've been there, and I can go there. It's going to be scary. But I will also get you out of there.

Much of the suffering of major illness, patients tell us, comes from the isolation—from a sense of being untouchable, of being beyond help, beyond care, beyond hope. The courage and fidelity of the companion become here just as important as his or her technical skill and knowledge.

We turn now to the last of our identified core skills—*Share authority* and *Be committed*. For most patients, healing is not complete when the time comes to leave the bounded container of the health-care system and cross once more through liminal space back into the "profane" world. This transit, like the one into the container, is fraught with peril and difficulty. Will the return to the ordinary harm the patient? Will the patient's return harm his or her family or community? Will there be "contamination" of one kind or another? Will the "exit" end quickly or be unsuccessful, necessitating a quick return to the healthcare container? Support for the patient becomes critical as he or she is released from the extra-ordinary encounter with the practitioner and is exiting the container to return to the ordinary world.

> Part of it is providing a plan to a patient that is logical to them. For some patients it's really easy. It's easy to provide a logical plan for the emeritus professor. It could be challenged, and they're, well . . . I have a couple patients that I know are absolutely brilliant. You don't need to have a medical degree to realize whether or not the plan your physician has set forth is logical or not. And I have patients that are really challenging. It is almost like a chess match with some of these patients.

The patient and the practitioner need to figure out how they will share in the treatment, the care that will go on once the patient is out of the practitioner's care and back into his or her own care and that of his or her family. Often this requires negotiation and a willingness to come up with creative options.

> I have to somehow come up not only with a treatment plan, but that something that the patient hasn't used already, and if they have used it, I have to convince them that they used it in an ineffective way, and that we are going to try it again. I have to convince them that notifying me four weeks from now is an adequate trial. Or I have to convince them that we really need to use this for six weeks. "The only treatment for your disease takes six weeks to kick in. Don't be mad at me for that. I didn't do the research!" Then you try to find something that will work quicker, but that might not be a long-term solution. You just have to work with your patients.

For any plan to carry weight, the patient and the family have to have confidence that the practitioner will remain engaged and available.

Each of the eight skills, it must be kept in mind, will be engaged in different ways as caregivers are confronted with different patient situations at each of the three phases of this ritual passage. Patients may enter the precincts of health care in a variety of states. Some will be having acute episodes and will be seeking immediate solutions. Others may have chronic conditions and be seeking maintenance treatment or amelioration of their current symptoms. Some patients in both those classes will be seeing their particular practitioner for the first time, and others will be repeat patients. And these entries into the healthcare system may take place in a variety of settings: doctor's offices, clinics, emergency rooms, or hospital admittance areas. Likewise, the activities performed by practitioners "within the container" will range in intensity and degree of intrusiveness, from a few questions and a quick listen with the stethoscope to major heart or brain surgery. And, finally, exits from the container are varied. Some patients with acute conditions will emerge healed, or on the way to health in short order. Others with acute or chronic conditions will be asked to return for additional visits. And some will exit the container by dying.

THE RITUAL STRUCTURE OF INTENSIVE CARE

We will look now at the details of an intensive care specialist's account of how he attends to and communicates about the transitions of his patients and their families. The intensive care unit (ICU) is one of the inner sanctums of biomedicine. Movements into it, activities and attitudes while within it, and exits from it are among the most charged any patient or family will experience. A particularly helpful aspect of the account that follows is the emphasis it puts on the practitioner's interactions with the families of patients. Too often discussions of biomedical health care overlook or diminish the role of families and the work they must do in the healing process of the patient. Even families that are absent wield enormous power, by their very absence. Part of the uniqueness of the ICU experience is the way it tends to bring the patient's family onto center stage. Here, too, ritual provides the best framework for appreciating the interaction.

Because I'm an intensivist, I usually work with families more than patients, in terms of the personal interactions, even though the clinical care is directed at the patient. So I've developed a strategy for establishing those relationships from day one, when a patient comes to the ICU. When I'm dealing with the patient initially, we're going to be in the survival phase, where we have an unstable patient. The case that comes to mind most readily with this is the traumatic brain injuries. Suppose I have a family who's been called to the hospital, and they know that their loved one was in a collision or is now on life support in the ICU with a traumatic brain injury, and they haven't seen him yet. And now I'm going to go talk to this family.

Day one is focused on the patient's survival, and on building a sound foundation for the intense relationship with the family such situations typically involve.

I introduce myself, and if they're willing, shake hands or whatever seems natural to do. And I understand that my investment at that first meeting is probably one of the most significant things I'm going to do as this moves down the line. What I do today is an investment in trust. And the most important trusting relationship in medicine is when it's time to discontinue life support and allow a loved one to die. The family and the patient need to trust that decision, and trust the person that's guiding them through this process.

There is almost always the special challenge that the practitioner has never met, much less worked with, this patient or this family before.

P (Practitioner): So my investment there on day one is the foundation that that trust is built on. That's why I need to know the easy things: the name, the gender. You know, they don't care about magnesium and all these other things—that's not what this is about. This is purely about whether their loved one is going to live or die.

I (Interviewer): Right. You mentioned body language, and you mentioned taking off your coat. I notice you now: you seem very relaxed. You're leaning back and . . . .

P: This is how I want to be to them, yeah. But that is often a major struggle, when you walk in to a group that's either hostile or upset.

In addition, there are pressures of time, and factors of enormous emotional and physical stress.

They think something's been handled poorly. Their loved one's now in the ICU because something bad happened in the operating room, something unexpected. And now I'm going to walk into that hostile environment. So I try to get comfortable and try to get to the point where they'll make eye contact. Some of them are so angry, they won't look at you, and I try to engage them. A lot of it is listening. I need to just acknowledge the fact that they're going to be going through this experience, and they need to know I'm comfortable with the experience, regardless of how horrible it is for them.

The fact that the practitioner has been here before shows itself early on as a critical resource for the patient. But this resource is only as valuable as it is reliable. Note also that certain words and phrases are layered in from the beginning. This is part of the orientation for the family to this strange and disconcerting container they are now entering with the patient and the physician.

P: And then I say, "We're going to do everything we know how to do, but they may or may not survive this." That's the take-home message from that first meeting. I want them to recognize that I'm going to tell them the truth. I always say, "I'm going to tell you the truth."

I: You say that very explicitly.

P: Yeah. "If I think he's going to die, I'm going to be telling you that." They need to hear the "die" word early on, if that's within the realm of possibility. Sometimes I'll say: "Chances are he won't survive this. Most patients with this type of injury die from it. I'm not saying that's what's going to happen, because it's too early for me to tell you that. But you need to be prepared. That's usually what happens here."

I: And you become trustworthy by virtue of the truth.

P: I will tell them—I say, "I'm going to tell you the truth, no matter how ugly it is." But I say, "You'll do better with the truth, and we'll be talking about the same thing." And consistently I hear them say, "Don't sugarcoat it. We want to know what's going on." They're searching for the truth. They can deal with the truth.

The truth answers a fundamental need. And part of it is that the truth confirms and supports the family's initial reactions and perceptions as family members try to make sense of the surrounding strangeness.

P: And I've already validated their fear that the worst thing they could imagine could happen here. So there's nothing lost in saying that, is there? I mean, it's a matter—see, it's a patient here on life support. To them, it looks like this is a person who could die.

I: It sure does.

P: "I've done this for twenty years. You're right. This is a person who could die." At the first meeting, I want them to understand that this is the survival phase—that either he'll survive or he won't. If he survives, there may or may not be other problems to deal with. But right now, we're in this survival mode. And then I tell them, "We're going to talk as often as we need to. I'm here, or my team is here, around the clock."

I: This is a message about availability.

The family and the patient will not be abandoned here in this often terrifying place.

P: Yeah. "We're here. And you're going to have questions, and when we get to this room, you may not remember. Some people find it helpful to write them down. I won't have all the answers, but I will listen to every question." And then I try to humanize the process for them, because a person may end up dying, and the language that I need at that point—I need to plant those seeds on day one.

Day one has involved a survival assessment and initial treatment, and taking the time to build a sound working relationship with the family. The interactions with the family have included careful attention to vocabulary—to terms and phrases that will be of increasing importance as the days in the ICU go on. With this, the entry phase is complete. We continue now to follow as the strategy for the next days unfolds, the days that will be spent inside the ICU container.

So that's the first meeting, which may take a half an hour, but I want them to have the time to ask the questions. The next time I meet with them, you know, once again, I want to try to sit down and go over things. But what I find is that if I spent the time up front, I get to the point where we can pass each other in the hallway and exchange ten or fifteen seconds' worth of communication, and they feel like they know everything they need to know about what's going on, because they don't have to worry that there's a piece of this I'm not telling them.

In the visits that follow that first one, I've found it helpful to ask what they're seeing. "I want to make sure that I answer your questions, and sometimes it's helpful for me to tell you what you're seeing."

The visual aspect of the overwhelming ICU experience is so significant that it is singled out for direct address. It also serves as a way to approach complex emotional issues in an initially neutral fashion.

Over the years, what I've learned is that they're seeing the very same things we are, but through different eyes. "Well, we see that he's swollen." Actually, that's one of the most common things I hear. And the reason I don't spend a lot of time talking about magnesium or basal pressures or anything like that anymore is because the time I've spent talking about that, they've been very polite and have listened, but at the end, they have one question: "Why is he so puffy?" I don't waste anybody's time talking about stuff that I'm interested in, because it's the practice of medicine but has very little bearing on what their experience is—and on how we guide them, or they guide me, through the process.

Note the use, again, of the word "guide." And of the acknowledgment that the family and patient guide the caregiver, as the caregiver guides them. Patient, family, and practitioner all have knowledge and skills that will be needed as this passage is accomplished.

> I: So the idea is responding to their concerns and their experience, as opposed to trying to guess what that might be, or tell them your perception of things.
>
> P: Um-hmm. Often, they'll say, "There are more machines in the room." "There are more alarms going off." "I see more IV bags." And I say, "That's what we're seeing, too. And that's because this is what's going on." What I find is that it's a validation of them when they realize that we're seeing the same thing they are. I want to get them in sync with why they're seeing what they're seeing. Sometimes they're saying, "We see now this isn't going on. Maybe things are getting better." And it's nice when I have a chance to say, "The reason that that's not there anymore is he doesn't need it anymore. I don't want to be overly optimistic, but that's one of the things we see in patients that are getting better."

The talk about the "visuals" continues to provide a place to begin conversation. And to be a place where information about prognosis and hopes and fears can be passed back and forth in manageable form. The underlying dynamic, which the practitioner is constantly intentional about, is trust-building.

> Sometimes, the first meeting, you don't even establish trust, but you have to be persistent with it. I mean, you can't shy away from these families. You're going to spend the time with them sooner or later. And it takes less time if you invest up front, because when it's time to turn things off, and that's when you're first trying to establish your relationship of trust, you're way behind the eight ball then.

If the patient begins to move more clearly towards death, a major shift in the relationship between practitioner and family must occur. This is where the family stands most acutely in need of a guide. It is typically the most frightening and most unfamiliar territory.

> P: We had a patient in the CV ICU where—this was one of those times where it almost was like following a script—and I pretty much knew that we weren't going to survive this. And so I talked to his wife about what we still had to offer. And we walked through those things in two days, and she saw this: that we did everything that was there to do. I don't want her to feel responsible for the decision that ended her husband's life. They have that sense—there's a tremendous guilt that they can carry for having made that decision. And so it's my responsibility to guide them through this. I've been there before; they haven't.
>
> I: Yes. That's right.
>
> P: And for me to put them in this position, you know: "What do you want us to do?" That's really an unfair thing. I told her, "This is what we have available to do. It may or may not work." And I had said before, "He may or may not survive this, and when I think he isn't going to, and when I think that what we're doing isn't going to change the outcome, or that we shouldn't go further, I'm going to be saying that." And when I tell them that, often, there's this visible sense of relief that they're not going to have to do this.

Once more, it is the matter of having been there before that is, for the family, the decisive aspect of the practitioner's expertise. Figure chart 2.2 the progress of the patient and the family through the ICU container. Notice the key themes in each phase and the skills needed to guide "novices" through the necessary transitions.

Training in biomedicine is not the critical piece at this utterly decisive juncture. Or, rather, that training is of importance at this juncture because it validates or "licenses" the guide to serve as guide. But the skills needed to help the families find their way are not part of biomedicine or of training in biomedicine.

And the day came that we'd rounded in ICU and the team acknowledged that it was time to quit. So I said to his wife, "After rounds, I'll come back and talk." And when I went back, she had asked her daughter to come in, and she said, "It's time, isn't it?" Which was what I was coming to tell her. So the idea is that if you really work together on this, you can be in sync. And the next question usually is, "How does this happen?" What they want to know is that he's not going to suffer. They want my assurance, and so I set that assurance for them early on. "The most important for me is that I keep him comfortable during this." This comes up frequently. You know, they see all this stuff going on and they can't imagine that he's not hurting.

New questions, new hopes and fears, new goals and priorities arise as the patient, family, and practitioner progress into the exit phase and prepare for the patient and the family to leave the ICU container.

P: So I'll go over the various medications: "These are two that are for his comfort. If he needs more, we give him more." And now I say, "The only thing we have left to do that is appropriate for him is to keep him comfortable. So all these things over here—we're going to turn off these things. But we're going to make sure that if we're going to make a mistake here, in terms of the administration of comfort medication, it's going to be that he got more than was necessary, and not less."

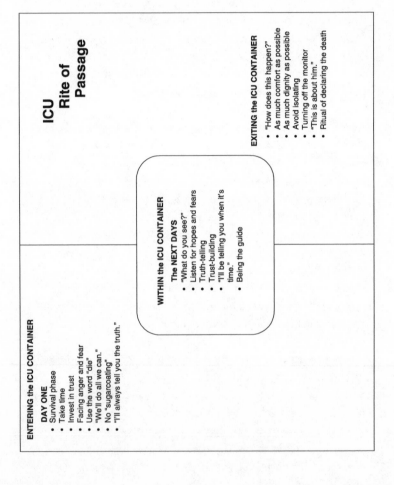

ICU
Rite of
Passage

ENTERING the ICU CONTAINER

DAY ONE
- Survival phase
- Take time
- Invest in trust
- Facing anger and fear
- Use the word "die."
- "We'll do all we can."
- No "sugarcoating"
- "I'll always tell you the truth."

WITHIN the ICU CONTAINER

The NEXT DAYS
- "What do you see?"
- Listen for hopes and fears
- Truth-telling
- Trust-building
- "I'll be telling you when it's time."
- Being the guide

EXITING the ICU CONTAINER
- "How does this happen?"
- As much comfort as possible
- As much dignity as possible
- Avoid isolating
- Turning off the monitor
- "This is about him."
- Ritual of declaring the death

Figure 2.2

I: Um-hmm. Not less.

P: Yeah. And often, they want to be at the bed side, because they want to be talking to him and holding his hand, and those things that might be comforting to him should he be able to perceive what's going on. Which, usually, they aren't. But, once again, if we're going to make a mistake, it needs to be on the side of comfort and dignity, as opposed to having somebody dying in isolation and pain.

There is renewed attention at this point to the power of visual impacts to shape the family's experience.

P: And then I turn off all the monitors, too. Over the weeks they've been in the ICU, families get focused on the lines and numbers on the monitor. If anything stays up there, it'll just be the electrocardiogram and the rhythm strip. "This just needs to be about how he looks; not about the monitor. You need to be looking at him, talking to him, and not watching the monitor. You know, this is about him."

I: Right. You change the focus.

P: Yes. And the focus is not on what we can do to keep the monitor running. The focus is on how comfortable he looks at the end of his life. And so then we sit at the desk, and we see on the monitor out there that he's flatlined.

The practitioner shifts here to describe something he learned from ICU nurses in his early days as a physician.

And then the nurses would say, "You need to pronounce him dead." And I'd say, "Is there some question?" But there is a certain process or expectation that allows closure. For me to say, "Yes, he's dead." And so the nurse would ask the family to leave, and we would go and close the curtain and I'd say, "We need to stand close enough so that they can see our feet under the bed, and we're going to stand at the bedside." So they see that there is some process going on here to make the declaration of death.

Another profoundly archaic ritual movement is taking place here. There is the ancient fear of abandoning or even burying those who are still living. And there is the matter of making sure that the dead are truly dead, and will remain on the other side of the boundary marking life and death. Both must be addressed. And simply looking at machines and monitors is not sufficient.

> And, ordinarily, we will listen for heart tones and check for responsiveness in someone that we know is dead. But there is some part of that doctor–patient relationship that's not closed until I've done whatever it is to verify once again that they're seeing what I'm seeing, and that in fact he is dead. Then I can open the curtain and go out and say, "As you know, Joe died, and the time of death is this, and I'm sorry for your loss. Are there questions that we can answer, or anything that we can do for you?" But short of that, it's not finished. There was a time when I thought it was, but the nurses said, "No, your job's not done here yet." Because it really is . . . it is a piece of it that, to me, is almost a myth, or unnecessary, or whatever, but for some reason, it's not finished until I've said it.
>
> I: Yes. Yes. I think it's like a ritual requirement.
> P: It is. Part of the ritual of death.

The technology and the science that claim the core of biomedicine do not answer, cannot answer, and should not be expected to answer these utterly fundamental needs and impulses of human beings faced with the end of life.

PRAGMATICS: THE "CASH VALUE" OF RITUAL

Our material suggests that extraordinary practitioners are aware of the ritual structure of key transitions involved in moving patients and families in and out of the various precincts of a healthcare system.

These practitioners recognize the need to prepare themselves and their patients for these transitions before they occur. They also recognize the need to attend carefully to the transitions as they unfold, and then come to completion. It is true that only a few of our practitioners frame these movements explicitly in terms of ritual. Yet their mastery of the skills needed to accomplish the critical ritual transactions involved in healing is clear. One question for further research, among dozens that suggest themselves here, is whether clinicians in a variety of modalities can increase effectiveness by consciously attending to, and taking advantage of, the fundamental structures of ritual as they seek healing for their patients.

Medicine itself as practiced from the beginnings of human culture by shamans, priests, medicine men and women, herbalists, and sorcerers has always been associated with ritual practices.[5] Even so, the question of how ritual might play a role in healing, if indeed it does, has vexed researchers and practitioners of allopathic medicine from its inception. Likewise, approaching the matter from another direction, anthropology has struggled with its own version of these questions from its very beginnings. And the young field of medical anthropology has inherited the quandaries of its elders. Thus a complex debate now rages in a variety of disciplines around ritual healing, symbolic healing, varieties of rationality, cross-cultural therapeutic effectiveness, and the relationship of all the aforementioned to the so-called placebo effect.[6] This newer version of the old debate, because it includes biomedicine as a full partner—biomedicine as theory, research program, and practice—carries a practical urgency that the classic discussions of science, magic, and religion did not.

Fortunately, we are not called on to take a position in this debate on the how and why of ritual in healing. The bottom line for us here, the "cash value," in William James's felicitous phrase, lies in exploring the pragmatism that characterizes clinical rationality.

[3]

HOW HEALING HAPPENS:
REPORTS FROM THE FIELD

Healing is multifaceted and multilayered. I'm more interested at this point in life in people being whole than being well. I think that true wellness is wholeness, and that really means that there is an acceptance of life, an acceptance of each other, and a desire to be connected.

One of the things that I believe very strongly is that healing is not equal to the absence of disease. If we think that, and we think narrowly that only if we can eradicate disease can we achieve healing, then we are again short-changing our patients.

We begin with two statements from two different practitioners, and we find two approaches to healing. Talking with clinicians, one gathers very quickly that an inquiry seeking a definition or, indeed, any single conception of healing is going to be fruitless. And, furthermore, such a project is quite likely to blind the investigators to the incredible richness of healing practices, the subtleties of healing skills that inform the work of the best practitioners hour by hour, even minute by minute, as they interact with their patients.

Healing is, as many of our interviewees stressed, a multifaceted, multilayered set of phenomena. At a most basic level, what is healing in one situation is not in another, or is harmful in another, or is simply irrelevant in another. Beyond that, many patients, indeed most all of us, bring to practitioners a need for more than one kind, or level, or layer of healing. Grief, for instance, accompanies any serious illness or injury. In turn, untreated depression can initiate a series of other problems, including poor nutrition, inadequate exercise, and failure to follow medication regimens. And then there are syndromes, like AIDS, or chronic conditions, like high blood pressure or diabetes, that manifest as illnesses in need of healing in a number of body systems. Every single interaction between practitioner and patient presents multiple opportunities for healing.

Likewise, each practitioner brings into patient interactions a set of therapeutic skills. Clearly, not all practitioners carry all skills, and no practitioner is limited to only one set. So the avenues for healing open to a patient are in part determined by the skill set of the practitioner. And this, in turn, hinges to a considerable degree on how the practitioner understands healing, and understands how healing occurs. Yet our interviews show that what is operational in practice is not a definition of healing—and only very seldom a systematic, theoretical approach to healing. What we consistently found were "clusters" of guiding notions that tended to be expressed in vignettes, anecdotes, brief stories, and autobiographical snippets.

In Chapter 1 we distilled interviews with 50 practitioners into eight essential skills, drawing general conclusions from a wide range of responses. In this chapter we will explore in detail one practitioner's "cluster" of responses to questions about how healing happens, and how one recognizes that healing has happened. The practitioner in this case (JM) began his career in family medicine and had a practice that included a significant amount of obstetric experience. As his career progressed, for reasons he explains in the interview, he began gradually to shift the bulk of his practice to end-of-life care. We have chosen to focus on this particular interview in considerable detail because its unusual range provides, in effect, an overview of healing that will be relevant to the daily engagements with patients of many kinds of caregivers.

We have also placed comments, explanations, and illustrations offered by other practitioners in boxes along the way. These selections are meant to elucidate the material in our primary interview and to provide the reader with a sampling of viewpoints and approaches, of modalities and specialties found in the broad range of our interviews. Sometimes this material will suggest a different point of view from the one found in our central interview. At other times, it will be a modification, a variation, a confirmation, a complement, or a warning. It is our intention, as well, to use these excerpts to make this chapter relevant in a variety of situations for as wide a variety of caregivers as possible.

1) IN THE BEGINNING: "IT'S NOT BECAUSE I'VE GOT THIS ASTOUNDING DEPTH OF MEDICAL EXPERTISE—IT'S ALL ABOUT RELATIONSHIP"

What do caregivers do to make the patient, and the patient's family, want them present at what JM calls "the deep tipping moments of life"? It begins with the kinds of little things discussed in Chapter 1. And then there is a second phase in which the ongoing relationship is solidified and becomes more complex. And finally there is the payoff when the relationship already built makes that critical difference.

> I: We're really trying to study healing and how it occurs. How practitioners develop healing relationships and what are the ingredients in that, with the hope that we can distill something out of this that will be helpful for our curriculum here, and maybe other places. So thanks so much for being willing to talk to us.
>
> P: This excites me so much.
>
> I: Great.
>
> P: I'm interested in the whole process and what you hope to gain.
>
> I: Maybe a good place to start would be to talk about—as you reflect on your own practice—what are the sorts of things you really attempt to do when you are establishing a relationship with a patient—that you think are really conducive to the sort of relationship you want to have with them.

P: I believe that relationships in and of themselves are therapeutic and healing. If someone feels connected then you're miles ahead in terms of being able to effect some sort of positive result and impact on the patient. So it's really establishing a positive, unique relationship where the patient remembers you.

Not only is relationship understood as the basis of all healing work that is to come, it is depicted as healing in and of itself. The opportunity to build a relationship is part, and the very first part, of the therapy that is being offered. And then comes the list of little things we have become familiar with. But notice the sequence—touch, position, and *then* conversation. Establish the relationship through the body first, and by the placement of practitioner and patient in the room. As the contact of practitioner's body with patient's body will be a central feature of so many treatments, the emphasis placed on attention to touch and position is apposite.

Touch is an extremely important part of that—so walking in, shaking hands, hand on the shoulder. Those sorts of things are very, very important.

Someone comes in for the first time and they're sitting down and they're a little nervous or anxious because they have never met you before. What I found really helps is—there's a physical context in terms of communication—where you are, position and juxtaposition with the patient. Removing any barriers between you. Keeping eye level similar—you know, three to five feet. All these technical things that hopefully they're teaching you in physical diagnosis class that you do to *establish the physical context*.

And then once you establish the physical context, a lot of *open-ended questions*. Typically for a new patient I'm asking: What are you here for today? How can I help you today? And what I have found is the little personal, nonmedical things that let the patient know that you're interested in them as a person. So I'm glancing and I'm looking at last names: Are you related to so and so? I see that you live on _____ . Do you know so and so?

Or: Have you lived there long? Where are you from? And if there is a point of connection, I exploit that. Those sorts of things really begin to solidify a personal relationship that goes beyond just, "Yes, you have a cold, and I'm going to give you some recommendations for how to take care of whatever it is today."

The open-ended questions do more than initiate a relationship. They provide the essential foundation, that shared body of information, on which an ongoing relationship with the patient can be built.

Now, on the ongoing relationship: What I've found is that patients find validation in knowing that they have something to offer as well. When I was in family practice, I had longitudinal relationships I had developed with families. If I had a daughter of a family or a young lady who was a waitress at a restaurant, I would intentionally go to that restaurant. I would intentionally sit in her section to allow her to serve me. So that she would understand that there is something of value that she's giving back to me. If I'm going to a store and see that someone is a clerk there, I will intentionally solicit that relationship and to allow her to wait on me.

What I found is those sorts of relationships really . . . it's . . . the word "endearment" is a little bit strong, but it really solidifies an aspect of personal connection and loyalty. To be effective as a physician, your patients have to trust you. And there's nothing that solidifies that trust more than saying, "I value you as an individual. I value who you are, what you do, and what you contribute to my life." And because of that you can implicitly trust what I recommend.

In certain life-changing situations, however, an enormously powerful connection can be forged very quickly:

I remember many years ago I was standing in a Wendy's—we would go to Wendy's with the kids for lunch on Sundays after church.

Box 3.1

As trust is being built, a structure of shared belief is also being put in place. Both patient and practitioner must believe in the practitioner's ability to heal:

I think, honestly, the first step in really healing the patient is to be confident. And that has to do with the way you interact, the way you speak about options, the confidence that you have in your own skills.

And both must believe in the patient's power to change:

It's all about trying to bring them to a certain state—to be able to receive some healing is really critical, really critical. So in the first consultation . . . that's my mission—to ascertain whether they're really ready to experience some healing.

Building relationship thus entails exploring the shared beliefs of patient and practitioner, and coming to an agreement about how healing can happen:

But where I think the healing really is, is opening to the possibility that we can actually change the system. Most people I see who have strong, catastrophic types of illnesses, cancers and things like that, tend to have such a negative view of the possibilities that there's no chance for healing. . . . When people can suspend their belief in that negative outcome, healing can take place.

A lady came up to me and said, "Dr. M?" That's not unusual because it's not a big town. What was unusual was that I had no idea who this person was. And she says, "Hi and so and so . . . "—and not a clue, not a clue. It turns out that I had delivered her baby when I was a resident. This was a dozen years ago. And I'd spent four or five hours with her.

But when I was doing my rotations, I attended my patients. I was in the room with them. I was observing them. I was watching them. And I was holding hands. . . . When I had a patient that I was assigned, I attended them. I delivered the baby, and then of course I never saw them again. That was it. They were in the hospital, and that's it. They were not my patients. I was just a resident. But as far as she was concerned, I was the person— forget the chief OB resident, forget the attending—I was the one responsible for bringing that life into the world. She never forgot; she never forgot. *Patients will remember you for who you were, not what you did.*

The practitioner–patient relationship, once "solidified," can broaden dramatically to become a place where practitioner and patient can meet and move together into "the deep tipping moments" of life.

What I find is . . . I just got an e-mail on Friday . . . and had an extended discussion with a former patient of mine, a young lady—she is probably 40ish—she has 6 kids. I delivered most of them. But 6 weeks ago she was having some chest pain. She had studies done—and she has a mass in her chest. It turns out to be a fairly rare type of cancer. But she has her medical care system set in place. One of my former partners is her family doctor, an excellent clinician. And her husband is a physician. They're very well connected in the medical community. But she called *me*. Because she had all these questions: What do we do now? How do I deal with this? God gave us these 6 kids, and now I have this disease. How am I supposed to handle this? What does this mean? She's having this existential crisis. She called me because she wants me to walk her through that process. She has excellent people. But what I found is that a lot of people don't necessarily, as physicians, develop a personal connection with their patients. So when it really comes to some of *the deep tipping moments of life*, their patients may not feel as comfortable approaching them.

A key point is that this kind of exchange, which so many practitioners cite as the most meaningful part of their practice, rests on doing "the little things," on the relationship-building skills JM refers to above, and that we examined in detail in Chapter 1.

2) THE ROUTINE EXAM: "I JUST KEEP IT SIMPLE. THERE WERE 3 F'S: FITNESS, FORGIVENESS, AND FULFILLMENT"

Beyond symptoms and sickness, there is the larger matter of the patient being ill at ease. And one appropriate setting for delving into this is the "routine" physical exam, where no acute condition claims full attention. It is here that the practitioner and patient can often most easily and comfortably explore the multiple layers involved in health, healing, and wholeness.

> When I would have patients in for their routine health maintenance exams, I would try to encourage the broader expanse of thinking in terms of what really, truly constitutes health. And I would tell them, "I presume you're in here today for a routine physical." . . . "My suspicion is that you're here because you are interested in your health, not because something's wrong. You're living a pretty good-quality life right now, and you'd like to live as fully and completely as possible for as long as you can. Let me share some of the things that I've learned about that." I break it down into three different categories in terms of trying to achieve ultimate and optimum health in your life. I just keep it simple. There were 3 F's.
>
> The first one was the *fitness* piece. And that's what people go to the doctor for, things like diet, exercise, and sleep. Nothing magic, sexy, or creative about it. You got to eat healthy; you got to exercise; and you got to get adequate sleep. Now for most people coming to the doctor, that is pretty much where it stops. . . . But there are two other very important things.

Here we make the transition into JM's practical implementation of this remark made earlier in the interview: "I think that one of the other limitations that I see when people think about healing is that they only think of it in the physical sense." Often we find the assumption that formulations of healing as multifaceted are relevant only to end-of-life situations or to lives majorly altered by debilitating traumas. The subtext is: Only when there is a failure to restore the body's functionality is there a need to address multiple layers of healing. But here, to the contrary, we see how one person brings a multifaceted conception of healing into his daily practice.

> The second F is *forgiveness*. People who are not willing to accept forgiveness from those they have hurt, and those who are not willing to offer forgiveness to those who have hurt them, will live with a burden on their soul, with an aspect of bitterness and emotional constraint that they cannot get rid of, and that no amount of exercise, sleep, and diet is going to overcome. So it's really important for us as individuals to make sure that our slate is clean. And it has to be on an ongoing basis, because we're flawed human beings. We're going to hurt people at every turn in the road, and people are going to hurt us at every turn in the road. And if we choose to carry that burden, we will never be fully healthy.
>
> I: Like a Chinese saying, "If you seek revenge you should dig two graves."
>
> P: Exactly. When I would see people who looked physically all right, but their blood pressure is up. No reason your blood pressures should be up. Or they're coming in with maybe a little back pain, but didn't really injure themselves. Or recurring migraines, with no reason for that. When I'm seeing these little things that are out of sync, that's where I go first. Let's talk about relationships. Frequently it's parents, frequently it's spouses, frequently it's kids. It's all the important relationship in our lives, where we've been hurt and have failed to reconcile those things. We talk about what forgiveness really is, from both the giving and receiving part, and what you need to do to manage that.

Box 3.2

Midwives are in a unique position to see the direct relationship of forgiveness to the body:

Now, I didn't know these people at all—but he was trying to be sweet to her and nice to her, and she was biting his head off. When that happens, he was not emotionally or physically present during the pregnancy. And now here he is at the last minute trying to show he's a good guy, and she is still pissed.

But I'm feeling sorry for this guy, because she is really biting his head off. She had been four centimeters for hours, and so I check her again and she is still at four centimeters. I want to tell her that she is five, but then she is going to want six. You know, you can't lie about this. . . .

I said, "He is really trying to help you, and you're biting his head off. Is there something going on here?" And she started crying and I'm thinking, "Oh God, stick your foot in your mouth and suck on your toes. You know you just did it again."

She said, "Honey, I'm just scared." He said, "It's okay— I'll never leave you again." Bingo. He kissed her, and she had a contraction. My fingers were on her cervix and it went from four to eight.

The third "F" is *fulfilling your calling.* And the way I describe that is that we are all wired and engineered for something. We are all born with a very unique palette of gifts, talents, and skills. And we do best when we are doing what we are wired to do.

Many practitioners choose to speak of wholeness when moving into the territory JM approaches with his 3 F's, forgiveness and fulfillment. One said, "I think healing is . . . looking at the whole picture, looking at mind and body and soul. It's looking at where they are in life . . . " Or again: "I suppose I would fall back on the old term 'holistic' or 'holism.' Looking at healing as being representative of physical, emotional, spiritual aspects . . . a sense of being complete or whole . . . I would even say it might be peace." How powerful it is, and how much sense it makes, to address this encompassing sense of health and wellness in the context of the regular check-in called "the routine physical."

In my family practice, I have a slew of examples in which people were very, very conflicted. And when you talked with them about those issues, I explored where their heart was, and what their passion was. Why are they doing what they are doing? Is it because of what they were led to do, or was it because someone said you should do this. . . .

The first time I really was conscious of this was when I was in medical school and I was on call. I was talking to a resident who was delightful woman from India. She was very skilled and extraordinarily sad. And around two or three in the morning, a little tired, and maybe a little vulnerable, and we talked about it. I got this whole unfolding. She was in medicine because it was the expectation placed upon her by her community. She was tagged early on to do this. She had come to United States; she was married; she had two young kids. She was very skilled at what she did—it wasn't that she couldn't do it. But it was causing a profound depression because she was so out of sync.

I don't even remember exactly what I said to her at that point, but it was something like, "It sounds to me like you are not in the place where God really intends you to be." This was not a religious discussion. She was Hindu—our concepts of deity were vastly different. But she was thoughtful about that. And I never saw her again. I found out that she had in fact dropped out of the program. She was very happy—living in a different realm.

I see people who are miserable in their jobs. People who are just miserable in relationships. They are not doing what they are wired to do. And, again, I don't care how healthy you are from a physical perspective. I see this all the time, where people will in fact try to compensate for these other failings in life—either not being in their area of giftedness or passion, or not achieving forgiveness. You can go to any health club and see them out there working out because they are trying to compensate for that. They just don't feel well and are not functioning at peak performance. They say, "If I just would get on this diet drink, if I would just use this weight machine, if I would just run this race, then I can overcome this." I think it's critical to address all those before you really achieve full health.

I: Do people need, in your view, permission to think about this?

P: Absolutely.

I: About the fact that they may not be fulfilling whatever their calling and mission in life is?

P: It's more than permission. They need permission to think about it. But they need guidance through that process. So they

---

Box 3.3

At times, the role of the practitioner shifts to that of a guide—helping to lead patients where they need to go or where their life wants to take them:

For me, it's not so much that you have fixed the disease, but that, for a particular person and a particular problem, you've really done everything you can to address it medically, and address it on a personal level and an emotional level. To make the patient feel that they've had everything, possibly, that can be done. And that, to me, is what our role is. . . . You've got to meet the expectations of the patient. And then I think another thing is that *you need to take the patient where they need to go*. I really like that—and by taking them "where they need to go" I mean what they need medically, and where they need to go emotionally.

---

need to be prepared—and how do I help to walk them through? There are a number of different wonderful things that I will encourage people to read through and think through before they make any significant changes. But the bottom line is the same.

You're going to find in your medical school class—they're arriving second year—you're already seeing students that are just embracing this, and they are so locked into where they need to be—and others that are just miserable. Talented, skilled, brilliant kids who are not where they should be. And the problem is, that when you get trapped like that, to break away seems like failure. And who are they letting down and disappointing? Should they drop out after their second year, or even midway through?

I: The pressures to remain are enormous.

P: They are enormous. I have seen students intentionally fail.

I: "I have to have a way out."

P: "I tried. I really tried the best I could."

A colleague of mine was in neurosurgery. Skilled neurosurgeon—a miserable, skilled neurosurgeon. He's farming now. He gave up the neurosurgery practice. And he could not be happier. Loves getting down there in the dirt, getting his hands dirty. Yeah, I think it's great. And his family's delighted.

Box 3.4

Who leads into the fear?:

So I'm not at all afraid of going to those dark places, even though they might be. Usually people are. I am not afraid to go to those places. To feel very held in a metaphorical way, very held by someone else when you're going to a really scary place is an amazing experience. Makes you want more. Makes you want to go deeper.

Alignment with who you are, and with what is seeking to manifest itself through you. To hold this with optimal grace and balance.
And what an extraordinary gift to find someone who is able to move
through your dis-ease and open the path for your deeper healing.

3) ADDRESSING THE LAYERS: "YOU KNOW WHAT, DOC? THIS HAS BEEN THE BEST 6 WEEKS OF MY LIFE"

Every practitioner is presented from time to time with the patient who,
in one configuration or another, presents a plethora of difficulties,
some of which are acute. An immediate task, as we see in the example
below, is to persuade the patient that some immediate healing, if only
in the form of symptom relief and control, is possible. Success on that
level makes possible conversation intended to persuade the patient
that additional layers of healing—including emotional, psychological,
and spiritual—are not only desirable but truly possible.

This is a young man who was in his mid-20s that I was asked to
see in the ER in the early 1990s. I was covering panel on that
particular day, which means that I was responsible for anybody
who came in unassigned to this small-town hospital. So they
called and said, "We got this guy down here that doesn't have a
doctor and he needs to be admitted. Come on down." So I did. The
kid had end-stage AIDS. We're a small town; we didn't see much
AIDS. And when we did, we didn't know what to do with it. To
this day, the most miserable human being I've ever seen. His
body was totally wasted by this disease. He was drawn, his eyes
sunken. He had fungi and sores all over his body. And he was in
exquisite pain. He couldn't breathe without pain. He would take
an inspiration, and he would shudder because it hurt to breathe.
And he would exhale, and it would hurt to exhale. Every breath
he was shuddering because it hurt so badly. And intractable
nausea, vomiting, and diarrhea. Bilateral infections in his lungs,

and his kidneys were all infected. He just was a mess. And, to top it off, he was just an incorrigible son of a gun. He was oppositional. He was defiant. He was angry. He was nasty. He had alienated everybody in his world. This is why he was unassigned. His health professional had pretty much abandoned him, as had his family and his friends. He really was there in his journey with nobody—and nothing in life, nothing.

He knew he was dying and his question to me was, "Doc, I just want the Kevorkian stuff. I know what's going on here. I can't survive much longer. I just need help getting out of here." And you really could hardly blame him. Here was a kid who was

---

Box 3.5

Who can be healed—and who fixed? Who wants to be healed—and who fixed? And how is the practitioner to make such distinctions on the spot?:

I: So not everybody can be helped.

P: Right, not everybody hears; not everybody is going to be fixed. Fixing again is separate—some people want to be fixed but not healed. They say, "Fix me. I want to get out of here." Most of the time they want to be touched. And they want to be healed most of the time, but not everybody. And that is where you go into this situation where there is a place for healing, even in this situation where you can't fix them.

I: It sounds like what you're saying is that we would have an impoverished notion about what healing is if we didn't acknowledge that it's a possibility all the time. Sometimes in really big ways, but sometimes in quite subtle and even routine ways, healing goes on.

absolutely miserable. He was dying. He had nothing, nobody. And I said, "I appreciate the extent of your suffering at this point. But I can't do that. That's against the law, and I prefer not to go to jail. But I think there might be some other ways that we can help you. So just give us a day or two." Symptom management was not difficult. We dealt with the pain, diarrhea, nausea stuff—that was quick—within a few hours at best to get them under control. And antibiotics for his infections. Dressings for the wounds. And, within a day or so, he physically was much more comfortable.

He was just as ugly and nasty as he was the day he came in. But at least physically he was more comfortable. He wanted to get out of there—and I said, "The only way I will let you out of here is if you go home with hospice, because you need somebody to be watching over you and taking care of walking you through these next days and weeks ahead." The nurse did a good job. She communicated with me on a regular basis. We kept his medications tweaked to make sure that he was symptom free.

I believe that this is a very important aspect of physical healing. Here is the hand you've been dealt—how well are you playing the cards? If you are playing the cards optimally for the hand that you've been dealt, then that's good health. When you have someone who is beleaguered by five diseases—MS, ALS, cancer and its complications—but you have them functioning at their peak capacity, that's health. We all have different physical limitations that are imposed by our genetics or conditioning or whatever, and our physical health is defined by our ability to function within the confines of those limitations. So physically, even though this AIDS was ravaging his body, physically we have the symptoms tuned up to the point where I'd thought he was physically healing—not physically *curing*, but physically *healing*.

The social worker then began working on trying to reconcile relationships. We found his mom, found his sibling, found a friend or two. They welcomed him back into their network. She began facilitating the reconciliation of these very damaged relationships. And so we began seeing healing on a relational basis—and

---

Box 3.6

Complex questions spring up rapidly when the role of persuasion in treatment comes into focus:

I: Another part of the healing process is actually convincing people to keep at it, to put up with something long enough. So that they can get, hopefully, the relief they want. A lot of this is persuasive, isn't it?

P: Oh yes, it really is. We talk about this in ecology of health care. What is the difference between persuasion, manipulation, and coercion? What we do in outlining this treatment plan . . . is being very persuasive, in the sense that you are going to enhance the benefits with words, and clarify or diminish the risk with either words or body language. "Yes, this medicine can damage your liver, but don't worry—I have never had a patient who had that problem." Or look the patient in the eye: "I can reassure you that with the labs that we are going to get every two weeks for the next two months, we will be able to detect any abnormality that might be going on." So that is the persuasion. That is the art of persuasion.

---

in the process, and then personally, on an emotional psychological basis. Healing was occurring as he was seeing some positive aspects in terms of who he was, how he felt, how he was reacting to his environment and to people in his sphere.

The chaplain got involved. This is a kid that, not unexpectedly, had long since abandoned the faith of his youth. The chaplain was able to walk him back to that and make that faith relevant in his current situation. Reconnect him with the God that he had previously honored and had known, and to really make his spiritual walk an important part of this process as well. So you saw this spiritual healing going on.

Whether one argues that connection defines healing, or that reconnecting is an essential component of healing, it is clear that patients improve when relationships with family and friends are repaired. And likewise, a compelling case can be made that patients do better when they can recover lost portions of themselves—whether it is a cherished and hard-won skill, a dark memory buried in shame, or a fundamental life passion. And all this should happen, for each of us, before death—or so argues JM.

> In every dimension this young man was healing. Physically, spiritually, emotionally, relationally, psychologically. I remember going up to visit him, which turned out to be just two or three days before he died. He looked up at me, and he said, "You know what, Doc? This has been the best six weeks of my life." And he died whole. He died healthy.
>
> I think about what would have happened if he had just been admitted and someone had narcotized him to the point of putting him in a sedative semi-comatose state. He would have died in a few days. Everyone would have said, "Whew, what a great relief," never having given him the opportunity to heal. Had he gone to a nursing home, would they have provided the resources that he needed to negotiate that kind of healing process? So one of my passions is that everybody have the opportunity to experience healing before they die.

There are, then, multiple layers or dimensions of healing to be addressed before one dies. And then there is the meaning of illness and health in each of those layers in the context of the patient's larger life story. Another practitioner utilizes a three-layer framework.

> I would fall back on the old term "holistic." . . . Looking at healing as being representative of physical, emotional, spiritual . . . it's a sense of not so much of being complete or whole as it is . . . I would even say it might be peace. A sense of peace about who I am, what my medical condition is, and what my condition means.

The stress she places on the word "peace" brings forward the element of assent to the realities of one's condition. Patients can alter their sense of the meaning of their medical condition. So one way to think of healing would be to consider it as the acceptance of a new vision of one's own wholeness. Thus one might have a medical condition that is certainly terminal, and yet be at peace with that, and come thereby into a place of healing.

4) END OF LIFE: "SHE HAD LONG SINCE PROVEN PHYSIOLOGY A WEAK SISTER WHEN IT COMES TO THE OTHER COMPONENTS OF OUR BEING"

Death is a preoccupation of all cultures—and, as horizon and as event, a force shaping all of our days. Healthcare practitioners have the privileges, the challenges, and the responsibilities of working in close proximity to death, or the possibility of dying on a daily basis. Listening to our caregivers report on their experiences accompanying dying people, we were struck again and again by what might be best described as the startling intimacy of death.

The initiation into healthcare work often comes through and by intimacy with the dead. Think of the relationship the medical student develops with the first cadaver. Think of what is learned and who the teacher is. Think of the intimacy of the scalpel in the relationship of hands—the student's hands—and those of the dead. And then there is the moment when a hospice worker first washes the body of a person he or she has been caring for days, perhaps weeks. No matter what has transpired between them, this further step into the mystery of dying is more intimate still.

Stories about the movement into death have ever been central for our understanding of ourselves as human beings. And among the most powerful of all are stories about death that are likewise stories of healing.

Box 3.7

"Death as Healing." This is a regular theme in our interviews. Yet one practitioner proffers a caution:

In the Jewish prayer for healing . . . the request is for healing of body and spirit, with the recognition that your body may not get healed, but your spirit may. And I like to see it that way—there's lots of ways a person can be healed. All of that said, I find that language just does not go over very well.

It's the mantra for a lot of people in hospice and elsewhere . . . but the truth is when you're walking the wards of _____ Hospital, and all these people who have come from far away for the cure . . . it just doesn't get you very far. And so I tend not to use that language very much. Sometimes, if I hear somebody talking about healing, I will say, "What do you mean by healing? What does healing mean for you?"

A mid-80s lady was admitted to our inpatient unit with advanced GI cancer. There was no treatment, and she didn't want it anyway. She progressed as expected, and she got to the point where she had stopped taking food or liquids. And then she lapsed into an actively dying phase. Breathing dramatically changed, maybe four times a minute. No longer conscious, no longer able to respond at all. Urine output dropped to virtually nothing. Blood pressure dropped very measurably—and when that happens, typically we have two or three days left.

I had a very frank talk with the son and grandson, and they wanted to be at the bedside when she takes her last breath. So two, three days passed—four days come, five days passed. We got a week out into the process, and the family was becoming exhausted, because they were not sleeping, not eating, and getting impatient and angry. The grandson says—actually that was my very first request for active euthanasia—"Please give her something. Put her out of her misery." I said, "The best that I can determine, she's not suffering at all. Let's talk about what we need to help you with your misery. But she's doing okay."

This went on a week, a week and a half, then two weeks. Defying physiology. We were at a month of not having so much as a drop of water, and yet her heart was beating, barely. No palpable blood pressure. But if you watched, every fifteen seconds her chest rose. She was still breathing. She was still there, a little hypothermal, but she still had a temperature. And throughout this process we were doing the things that hospice people do in terms of readiness: Did she make peace with people? Is she right with God? The family had given her permission to go.

So all this stuff was being done—two and half weeks out in this sequence, which should have lasted two days. Then a friend of the family came in. She nudged me and said, "What's going on?" I said, "I don't know. She won't die. Maybe you can help." We went through the same sequence of questions. She said, "You know she has a daughter. They parted 25 years ago. They'd had some disagreements, and then parted, and it wasn't all that favorable." I wondered whether they could resolve it, even though they have not spoken to each other in 25 years, and I said, "Do you have any way of getting ahold of her?" She replied, "I haven't had any contact with her in maybe 10 years, but here is the number I have."

So I walked in the room, and I called from the bedside phone. A lady answered the phone. I said, "This is the doctor from hospice. Is this so-and-so?" "Yes." "I am so glad to be able to get you. I just want you to know that I have been taking care of your mom. She developed cancer some months ago, and she has been declining ever since. She is very close to the end of her life now. I just found out that you two had parted some years ago, perhaps not on the best of terms. I know in those circumstances some things can get left unsaid. Some things you might want to tell her and talk to

---

Box 3.8

Death as healing at the end of life, yes. But where, one may ask, is the healing in the death of a child?:

I had a child dying of a brain tumor. I had told him and the parents good-bye that morning, and he died later that afternoon. I had to go over and pronounce the death, but I didn't rush or hurry, because I knew the parents well, and we had already taken care of all that. We got there maybe a couple hours later, and everything was out of the room except the boy's body, and the bed had been stripped. The male nurse and I stood by the bed-side. He shed a few tears, and I said a prayer—and then I can remember this incredible, absolutely incredible sense of peace. And I thought about that so often, but then I realized that the peace came from the realization of the wholeness of that child who died totally and completely unaffected by the great worries of the world. He died totally, totally whole—and that is an awesome thing to realize.

---

her about." She said, "Well, yeah." I said, "You need to understand that she is very close to the end of life. She is not responsive at all. But I am going to put the phone up to her ear to give you a chance just to say whatever you think you might want to say to her. I don't know if she can physically hear you. But I think she will know that you are there." So I put the phone down by the patient's ear. I can hear chattering—kind of wanted a speaker button. What do you say to somebody after twenty-five years?

After about five minutes, I see tears rolling down this lady's face. It was a very powerful moment—because logically, where is the substrate for this? She has no water in her body. Obviously this had nothing to do with physiology—zero. She had long since proven physiology a weak sister when it comes to the other components of our being. You want to know what's really powerful in life—it ain't physiology or biology.

So the tears were streaming down her face. I heard the chattering stop, and I took the phone back and described to her daughter what I just saw. "I want you to know that she heard what you said, and that her tears flowed. This is a very healing process for her. I thank you very much." I hung up the phone—and five minutes later she was dead. Clearly there was something she needed to complete in her journey toward health. She was not going to die until it was done. People don't die until their lives are complete.

Death as completion—and completion as one criterion of healing, and of a healthy life. Our interviews indicate that this perspective is shared by practitioners across disciplines and traditions, as this excerpt from an interview with an acupuncturist suggests:

P: I remember how profound it was when my teacher said, "Healing isn't necessarily about getting well." I feel like what I've been doing my whole life is healing. And so in my healing process, I am affected by my patients who come in, and they are affected by me. We are, in essence, helping each other heal.

I: I volunteered in hospice for years—so the idea that "healing may not mean getting well" makes complete sense.

P: It almost gives you permission to die, you know? Because you aren't feeling like giving up; you're feeling like you're just moving towards something else.

Again and again our practitioners bring forward these distinctions between "healing" and "getting well," "healing" and "curing," "healing" and "fixing." As one might expect, such discussion hovers all around their accounts of the dying process. These pairs of terms allow practitioners to describe that critical shift out of what many understand as an active approach to healing and into one that emphasizes presence. The ability to make this shift is a requirement for caregivers working

---

Box 3.9

What relieves the loneliness of dying?:

P: For many of these patients you're one of the most important people in this whole process, because they know you're there. You're kind of a safety net or safety blanket. "If you're hurting, I'll be here." "You need someone to talk to, I'll be here." Availability... just to know that they've got you... I think that's the real thing about dying—it's just the lonesomeness of it. The fact that no one is sharing it with you. You're all alone. Even though you've seen other people die it's... and there may be eight people in the room, but nobody else is dying right now.

I: You're going out by yourself.

P: It all comes down to a very singular experience for each of us. And some way of feeling like you're at least there... your presence... just, I think, you know, that's what touching and presence... a presence in the here and now, somebody you know... when you're taking care of them.

---

with the dying. Once more, JM has a moving story that illuminates this territory:

We had a situation just a couple of weeks ago, with a former employee at our hospice—one of our dear, dear sweet nurses. She was about 60 . . . just really was truly endearing. Loved by everybody she took care of and worked with. She had to stop working because of a heart issue a year or so ago. After that, she was diagnosed with cancer. She had always said that for her last days she wanted to be back with the people she used to work with to provide her care.

I got a call on a Monday. "I thought you might want to know that _____ just got here." "I'll be right over. How is she?"

"Well, she's agitated, and has no idea who she is or where she is."
Now she was as good to me as she had been to everybody else. We
had a very good relationship. When I arrived at the bedside she
was restless. She was thrashing around in the bed, and there were
staff people on either side trying to calm her and hold her just a
little bit so she wouldn't hurt herself. I walked over and one of the
staff members stepped aside, and I put my hand on her shoulder.
The nurses are saying a little loudly, "Dr. _____ is here." And she
didn't respond to that at all. So I reached down and kissed her
forehead. I said, "Welcome home _____." I stayed there for a
couple minutes and then left.

I heard later that that was the only thing that gave her peace.
Her nurse said I walked out of the room, and she immediately
calmed down. It was a very powerful acknowledgment of what
presence does—and the power of a relationship. Someone else
walking into that room and putting a hand on her shoulder and
saying, "Welcome home _____" would not have had the same
effect, because they didn't have the existential relationship
with her.

Yes, I could have pumped her full of Haldol and other drugs,
and eventually medicated her to the point of unconsciousness . . .
but presence and relationship—that's healing. That is healing.
One of the things that I believe very strongly is that healing is
not equal to the absence of disease.

Acknowledging presence and relationship as healing both entails,
and is entailed by, a conception of healing that is broader than the
absence of disease.

If we think narrowly that only if we can eradicate disease can we
achieve healing, then we are short-changing our patients.

This final comment prepares us for what most would consider
the far more radical stance one of our practitioners takes: "Healing?
When you can enter death as part of a process, without regret and

without fear." Healing as the work of an entire life—carried on by everyone who enters and exits that life, in each and every moment.

5) PRACTICING PRESENCE: "PRESENCE IS BEING WILLING TO BE LED, AND NOT FEELING LIKE YOU HAVE TO ORCHESTRATE . . ."

Presence, our practitioners agree, is not something that can be forced. It is not something that can be "done"—either "done to" or even "done for" another. As such, it is impossible to quantify and difficult to teach. And yet it is something patients recognize instantly.

> What you're going to find in your third-year clinical work, and many medical students do, is that the patients prefer the medical students over the residents and over the attendings. And that's because that student is the individual who sat down with them and spent time with them. Presence was a very powerful healing force, and patients recognized and wanted that.

As an acupuncturist succinctly puts it: "True human presence is itself healing." But granting that patients long for this quality in their caregivers, there is still the puzzle of how this can be offered, taught, described. Commenting further on the case of the hospice nurse examined earlier, JM explains how he makes his presence available to his patients.

> P: I was not intentionally going in saying, "What I am going to do is to heal _____ at this moment." That was just a spontaneous reaction on my part that I did with the intent of just fully embracing her and letting her know that I was there and that we were glad she was there. And yet it had a very positive, healing effect on her.
> I: The spontaneity, is that an important characteristic of it?

Box 3.10

One practitioner warns that broadening our conception of healing, wellness, and disease carries with it a danger:

P: But you have to end up not blaming the victim. I mean, that's one of the problems with some of the focus on good life and attitude, so that if you get cancer, then somehow or other . . .

I: "Obviously, I'm an idiot."

P: "You're an idiot. It must be your fault." "You did something, because if you were properly taking care of yourself, then this would not have happened." Or the person with cancer reads articles about people with good attitudes doing better—and if he's not doing better, that must mean that something is faulty about his attitude. So you've got to be careful to avoid that trap in a lot of different ways. Yeah. You can be healed and still die at the same time. That's one thing that people have a hard time getting their hands around.

I: Dying is part of the healing.

P: Well, I think that a lot of it can be intentional. A lot of it absolutely can be intentional. And when you start thinking in terms of that distinction between "presence" and "provision," again understanding that your presence is there being willing to be led, and not feeling like you have to orchestrate it.

Spontaneity here indicates that it is not the practitioner's agenda that is preeminent, not the doctor's priorities that dominate. Only if the caregiver is able to get outside his or her own concerns is this kind of healing response possible.

You can plan to be present, but you may not necessarily be able to plan what is going to unfold in those moments—because what the patient says, what the patient does, how the patient reacts, what the family members are going to ask you—you just simply have to be prepared to go with their flow, be intuitive enough to understand where their pain is coming from or their concerns lie, to be able to ask open-ended questions to allow them to process that.

Being truly present requires a willingness to remain undecided, a willingness to be open to opportunities that may appear suddenly, unexpectedly in a given setting.

I may not be able to help, but if they know I've listened to them, that I've heard, that I'm concerned and that I will get resources for them that will help them with whatever they put on the table, then they're happy with that. I think that one of the other limitations that I see when people think about healing is that they only think of it in the physical sense.

Pushing for yet another way into the question of presence and healing, JM explores a distinction between the terms "provision" and "presence" that he first heard made in a religious context:

A friend of mine is a singer and songwriter, and well known in the Christian music community. In the course of a series of lectures he noted that what we need from God is His presence and His provision. I have taken the same approach with understanding what patients come to us as physicians for. There are two things we have to offer, our presence and our provision. We are trained in the provision. That might mean to do surgery or provide a prescription. That is what patients come to us for, what we are trained to deliver. So patients come in expecting provision, but if they don't get that, somehow they feel like they've been short-changed. But what patients don't realize, and unfortunately most physicians don't understand, is that the presence is sometimes more powerful, more healing, more therapeutic than the provision.

Other practitioners speak here of a distinction between "expertise" and "presence." These more familiar terms can help us understand

---

Box 3.11

"Being a mirror" is one way of staying present:

I try to hold up a mirror for folks ... without judgment, holding up a mirror, without shame, without blaming. Just asking in some way or other, "Is this really what you want for your life in the deepest way? Or is there another way for you to get what you really want?" So that's another piece—helping people find through dialogue, and by just being present with them in a loving way. To find, "Well, what is it you really want? Because your life is expressing in this way, and it's not getting you what you want."

---

what JM means when he speaks of the distinction between "provision" and "presence." A urologist goes at it this way:

The greatest gift you give anybody is your presence, not in the verbal sense [talking], but just being present ... to sit down on their level and be quiet. That is a gift. It is the greatest gift I can give them. My expertise is not what my gift is. My gift is to be present; and then I help people.

And "presence" brings a reciprocal gift that "expertise" cannot:

And it [being present] is a beautiful thing, because it is such a privilege. Not many people get to do that. The privilege of being given the gift of another person to you. I get the gift of their lives to me. And you never cease to be amazed by that gift that you get by being there for somebody. They give me the gift of healing, and I give them back my presence. It is amazing how patients really understand that.

I: So this is the payoff?

P: The payoff is, "Thanks, Doc. I'm glad that we got to be together today."

This "gifting" back and forth is one of the fruits of cultivating relationship and presence as healing in and of themselves. A very important point, folded into this interaction, is that presence and relationship *heal the healer*. Put differently: A critical element of self-care for the practitioner is learning to develop relationships and to cultivate the capacity to be present. Presence is healing for both patient and caregiver.

But what is required for the willing practitioner to be able to sit still, to be open, to follow the patient? This inquiry drives the questioning deeper. To be present to the patient, the caregiver has to be able to escape his or her own story, to be skilled enough to transcend his or her own "hot buttons." Our practitioners come at this matter of getting beyond their own ego-projects and priorities from many different directions. One quotes a favorite author: "We undergo a slight but significant change in personality." Another points to a far more encompassing, even Herculean undertaking:

> P: It's more self-exploration so I can do clearing of my own crap. I clear my own stuff as much as I can.
>
> I: Okay.
>
> P: I've opened myself up in such a way that I can hear other people's stories, and not let my own stuff get in the way, and be very comfortable where they are. I don't have to have an agenda. I've done my own work. My ego is not the only one—that's very important to say.
>
> I: So it has its place. It's taken care of.
>
> P: That doesn't mean I don't catch myself. I have to catch myself because I am human, right? My ego will get in the way, and then I have done enough work to recognize, "Oh wow! My ego feels in the way." I'm getting frustrated with this person, and what am I going to do about it? So it is not that I don't ever feel it. It's that I do work to recognize it and do something with it, and get back through the person's story, not mine.

Being present to others requires being present to one's self—and being able to set that self's concerns aside. Healing others in the most fundamental ways requires significant, internal effort of practitioners as they strive for their own healing.

> P: The practitioner has to take it deeper through their own cultivation—self-cultivation.
> I: How has this new work in your own self-cultivation altered the way you receive new patients?
> P: The deeper I go into my path, the less need I have for others to share that path—the easier it is to accept others where they are.

To these classic images of clearing and cultivation others add religious imagery of surrender and emptiness. They speak here of the potentially enormous transformation a practitioner can undergo in the journey to be present and healing for others.

> There is no question that, over the years, the times I surrender are the most powerful times in people's healing process. What surrendering means may differ from moment to moment. But it's what you might describe as "not about me." It is not even about death. It's about being big—being—not just doing, but being. I heard years ago a quote from _____ . He said, "The most powerful part or influential thing in a human relationship or a healing of a person or patient is the consciousness of the doctor." And I believe that.

What is being described here is a state of being "bigger" than death. And, indeed, it is just such a state that our practitioners point to when they speak of death as healing, and healing as death—when death is entered "without fear and without regret." The import of the word "surrender" is, in part, its dramatization of the setting aside of core human fears that is necessary if one is about the business of "being big."

Thus the puzzle of presence brings us, by way of "surrender," back around to the qualities of being that are native to healers, back around to the quality of life of the practitioner. What kind of living makes it possible to surrender in situations that would seem to demand action, control, and "orchestration"?

I: These larger forces are supporting the healing movement—and inviting, opening doors and inviting, empowering all of us to go through those doors.

P: Exactly. I'm being carried. And I try to surrender to that all the time. . . . All the religions have a concept of this. In native traditions, they call it "becoming the hollow bone." And I know in Judaism, they talk about being the "empty vessel." It's that idea of clearing out—clearing out all your own places: your snags and snares, and things where emotions can get caught, feelings, fears, physical stuff; stagnancies can get caught and then grow in you as a practitioner. Trying to keep all that clear with cultivation.

Many of our practitioners emphasized that human healing takes place in an arena far, far greater than the human. Living in concert with these larger dynamics is another stance the verb "surrender" can indicate. The metaphors "emptying" and "becoming hollow" describe the feeling of having set self aside—the state of being cleared out. And it is that state that allows the practitioner to be present both to the patient and to the larger powers that encompass patient and practitioner alike.

But even as she speaks of surrender, this clinician refers as well to "snags" and "snares," "fears" and "stagnancies"—all words of danger. What is necessary for healers to avoid being made ill themselves as they move daily in the presence of illness? Another practitioner put it this way:

I think the one thing we have to do is this: *We have to practice life—not practice medicine, but practice life*. And practicing life to me means . . . it's like anything you practice. There's a routine to it. What do I do daily that is practice *in my life* for my life? My practice is partly physical. I do some yoga. I do meditation. I do some contemplation and reading.

There is the bodily practice of learning centering postures, and learning to be still. And there is cultivation of the mind, of awareness and the intellect. And then there is "the dance."

And then I think another thing that we have to practice is mindful listening. You tend not to listen because you get pressure and you want to move on. Your tendency is to break in after eighteen seconds . . . So mindful listening—and that means a practice. That means *every time you are with somebody you have to remember that, in this moment, I need to listen, not respond*.

You have to learn a dance. I'm stepping on your toes, and you're stepping on mine. But you've got to remember you're going to do that sometimes. You are going to step on some toes. You immediately think, "Well, it's time for me to speak," and then all of a sudden you know it's time to back off. "I just stepped on your toes. Sorry, go ahead." It's a fun thing to really try to do that. But that is the practice.

I: That's the practice.

P: Every day.

I: It sounds like such a fundamental skill. Are the meditation, yoga and the reading that you do . . . are those things that keep you in a place where this is possible to do, or do they deepen or enrich it? I am trying to see the connection.

The extrapolation that another clinician offers at this point is truly extraordinary:

P: What it allows you to do is to develop a rhythm of allowing yourself stillness and thought. Then when you go to do your work, that rhythm pervades what you do. If you can allow it to happen. But if you don't do the practice of allowing the rhythm to develop in you, then you never are able to get to the point of allowing that to happen with the things you do out in the real world.

I: That is great. So in a way it is a nurturing dimension of stillness which you can then transport into the patient.

A practiced, internalized rhythm results in that rhythm being carried out into the world. Thus one can "practice life" within one's

---

Box 3.12

"If you're truly a healer, you know early on."

I: Was there a kind of motivation that you came to this work with? Or did it develop in the process of becoming really skilled at what you do?

P: You can learn some skills to be a healer, but you have to be a certain kind of open person to be a healer. If you're truly a healer, you know early on. I mean, people will come to you with their stories when you are five.

I: Yes.

P: When I was twelve I was the one that people would just come to because I knew how to say it and be open, and I knew already. *I had the heart. I just didn't have a lot of technique.* So part of it was just how I was brought up and who I was. Part of it was—and this is true for a lot of therapists and healthcare providers in general—there was a lot of crap in my family, and I had the role of taking care of the crap. So I actually learned to channel that into an occupation. I already knew how to do it; I just wanted to do it really well. Part of it was that if I couldn't fully heal maybe my family, I was damn well going to heal other people. And that is very true for a lot of health providers.

I: Yeah.

P: So I think most of these things started early and then along the way became much bigger. And then further along the way it became, "I want this world to be a kinder place, and I'm going to do it." I can help that along. So I really love what I do. I can't imagine doing anything else.

---

own life in order to practice medicine well, no matter what modality or tradition informs one's clinical skills. And it is such a rhythm that can help keep things clear, help one move past the "snags" and "snares," help one become a healing presence.

6) THE HEALTHY PRACTITIONER: "I DON'T BELIEVE THAT ANYBODY IN THIS WORLD IS INDISPENSABLE"

Turning now from the cultivation of presence to the healing of the practitioner, we go back to JM as he talks about his own alignment and fulfillment. Other practitioners use the theological terms "calling" and "vocation" here. We will compare JM's ideas on this subject with those of a psychotherapist, in a linked series of adjacent boxes.

I remember I had a professor in medical school, who—actually I had worked with him before I got into medical school, in the physiology department, in the lab doing a lot of bench research—at the time, came to acknowledge and appreciate my research ability, my research skills. I told him I was going into family practice, and he just said, "What a waste. What an absolute waste of talent." And I thought, "Excuse me!"

I: "Thanks a lot." (Laughter)

P: "Yeah, I like working for you too, _____." But he was just so narrowly focused on, "This guy did good work for me, and he could do great work." And so he's wanting me to do an M.D./Ph.D., and he's got these different university settings. And here I want to be a family doctor.

I: That was your track.

P: That's what I was wired to do. And yet influential people can still, unwittingly, push people in directions that they think they should go.

I: Did you have significant mentors that taught you the things that you now know, both about establishing these relationships and sustaining them? Or are these things that you learned in your own practice, simply because you noticed that they work?

P: In terms of mentors, no, I didn't have anyone that was alongside me that I looked at and said, "I want to be like him." What I found was people in a reverse mentor role, "I don't want to be that way. I'm not finding that patients respond to that individual." Now, unfortunately, in our traditional medical setting,

---

Box 3.13

"Do you ask anyone why they do this? Why they want to be a healer?"

P: I have thought a lot about that this year, at difficult points. Why do you want to do this? Why am I doing this crazy thing?

I: Why am I doing this?

P: Why am I doing this crazy work? Why don't I just lie on the beach and play the ukulele? That would be fun. And the answer is, *Because I can't imagine any greater calling.* It's almost like the priesthood for me. It's not a job. It's a calling to give of oneself, of one's heart, fully to another human being. And doing that in the service of having them be open and be expansive. There is a ripple effect of what I do out of healing presence. Someone else gets that healing, and they become a healing presence, and it becomes a much more loving world. I see it in a really big way. I am but one person. But maybe that starts a wave of compassion and openness for a kinder world, and that is really important to me.

---

you are patterned to be like the people you're following around with the longer white coats . . . [the ones] that quickly leave and just kind of flutter out the window.

And so my plea to medical students—if you've heard me in any of the classroom settings, hopefully one of the things you did hear was that *our job is to treat people, not treat disease.* In our medical educational system the bias is more towards treatment. But if you think about the person and you regard them, honor them, and develop that relationship with them, they will never forget it. They will never forget it. It will be very powerful for them.

Many practitioners spoke of that very profound moment where all the world drops away and the caregiver and the patient are all that there is. These are moments of heightened perception, both physically and, if you will, "morally" or "spiritually." This intensity of connection in the sphere of vulnerability is a great part of the power JM speaks of above; and it is surely a most significant part of why others say plainly, "I can't imagine doing anything else."

I: Could you talk about some of the things that you do as a person to sustain your own sense of balance and wellness?

P: I love what I do and I love being with people, and so it's natural for me to stay late and to just kind of wander the halls and come in and sit with people and chat with them. It's amazing the number of providential encounters you have with family members. If you hadn't been there at that particular time, you wouldn't have had a chance to chat with family, learn this about the patient, or to be able to touch this particular need. And so I get very jazzed about that, and that's very meaningful. I think what I've been able to do, though, is to understand the importance of balance. I'm not letting anyone set that expectation for me. That's not something that I have locked myself into having to do for any other reason. If I need to leave early, I leave early. It's not that big a deal. But I know that earlier in my medical career a lot of my availability was because I felt an obligation to be there, to be the one—to be on call, to be available, to be this wonderful martyr—the self-sacrificing, dedicated physician. I felt that need. I felt so important and so valuable and valued.

I: (Laughter) It's a real high, isn't it?

P: Yeah, it is. And it's a dangerous one, too. It took some very good friends, and life circumstances, to knock my ego down a notch or two. This was very helpful. So I don't have preconceived notions of my own self-importance anymore.

A third practitioner underlines the importance of "very good friends," of having a "guide":

I think one other thing we don't do—and this has been my biggest failure as a physician in my years of practice . . . and that is not caring for the other caregivers as well as I should have.

Box 3.14

"Healers need other healers to help with the healing process."

I was holding a lot of stuff, not fully nurturing myself and always out there. Out, out, out—and then there is no time for nurturing and rebuilding. It's just always out, and then you're just tired—and then you're out again, and then you're tired. During a tired period . . . that is not a good time to be healing with anyone, because you're just empty.

And my guide helped me to understand the necessity of taking time off for rebuilding. And that that's not a failure. That it actually takes love and courage. It's a very self-loving, caretaking thing to do. But something I never learned how.

So I really appreciate an external person saying, "This is a good thing. Try it, even if it's uncomfortable. Because, one, it'll be a loving thing to do for yourself—and, two, you'll be a better healer if you do." Right, right. Kicking and screaming I went. Kicking and screaming.

I: Great.

P: Healers need other healers to help with the healing process. We have to have relationships with healers in order to be healers ourselves. I absolutely believe that. I have no doubt in my mind.

The intoxication of healing, the power that manifests as healing happens, is sometimes simply overwhelming for practitioner and patient alike. To keep in balance, to remain true to the fundamental calling, to stay aligned with what "you're wired to do"—this, finally, is impossible without healers healing the healers.

One way that balance, or the lack thereof, shows itself is in the practitioner's assessment of his or her own importance.

> P: You may or may not have heard yet that I'm leaving.
> I: No, I didn't know that.

HEALERS

P: They sent out letters just a week ago today. And someone said, "But you're indispensable." And I said, "No," and I argued that point vigorously. "I don't believe that anybody is indispensable." And he said, "Well, what I hear is that you don't want people to miss you or that you're not valuable." I said, "No, no, no—not that. I want people to miss me, and I want them to think fondly of me. But I want them to be better after I leave." I hear the word "indispensable" and the thought is that somehow things can't go on or things will be worse.

I: Things will go into the ditch, right?

P: Right, and I absolutely eschew that philosophy. I don't believe anybody in this world is indispensable. They create value, and they're integral to life. But earlier in my career I believed that I was indispensable in my own environment. And you know, if we're honest about those really secret things in our heart, we like to believe that people would never do as well without us.

I: (Laughter) Oh, yeah, right.

P: I heard this little blip from a musician that was involved in raising up talent. He did a great job of this over the years, and this comment really helped me in terms of how I viewed my own professional growth. He said, "You know, my job is to bring in people that do what I do, but do it better." I really like that. I really like that perspective. That's what I did in my practice. I brought eight partners into that practice. And I brought in people that I thought could do what I did, and embody some of the principles and the belief structures that I had, but that would do it better than I would.

"No one is indispensable." This can be an operating principle, as well as a truth, as JM makes clear. But some practitioners do stand out—as models, teachers, guides—as having remarkably refined skills, or prescience, or intuition. And it is they who make it possible for the ones who come after them to "do it better." Expertise is passed on to the next generation by richness of guidance and quality of insight. The capacity for healing is in part a matter of such expertise—but it is also a matter of gift and calling, as our practitioners have shown.

[4]

HEALING TRADITIONS: THE ROLE OF RELIGION AND SPIRITUALITY

Among the most fascinating contributions to our study were those offered when the conversation linked healing with religion and spirituality. This chapter is devoted to this complex and often controversial territory, and we will once more take our cue primarily from the interview material itself. It is, of course, no surprise that our caregivers had much to say about these matters. But what may be surprising is how little talk there was about beliefs and doctrines, and how concrete and action-oriented the talk was. As in earlier chapters, the emphasis here is on practices: "What do my patients do?" "What do I do?" "What can we do to help healing happen?" This emphasis on the "doing," the "how-to" or "pragmatics" of religion, will be our touchstone throughout this chapter.

Another striking feature of the responses was the range of discourse. A wide variety of words, terms, expressions, metaphors, and images were used to describe how religion and spirituality are related to healing. A small portion of this discourse was drawn from the vocabularies of major religious traditions, such as "the Gospels," "meditation," or "Qigong." But doctrinal, exegetical, theological, and confessional language appeared infrequently, and references to law and scripture almost never. What we mostly found were common everyday words, used in ordinary ways. "Compassion," "humility," "surrender," and "service" all bring recognizably religious and spiritual connotations alongside their "secular" meanings and usages. We heard no scientific explanations of the power of prayer, and very little theological explication of intercessory prayer. The talk was more on the order of, "Be compassionate, and people get better." "When people forgive, their health improves." "When people feel connected to larger reality, they find new energy for healing." This talk was all typically couched, as in earlier chapters, in vignettes, anecdotes, and stories, which were followed by suggestions, extrapolations, or instruction about what to do. "Some of my patients do this." "I've tried this." "Try that and see if it makes a difference."

The immediate questions that concerned our clinicians had little to do with asking, "Is there a role for religion? Is there a role for spirituality?" Their concerns were more likely to be:

- How appropriately to make room for the patient's religious belief
- How to make possible ongoing connection with a patient's religious community and his or her minister, counselor, teacher, rabbi, priest
- How to keep sound boundaries between a clinician's own religious belief or spiritual practice and that of their patients

This listing reflects clinical realities. In major medical centers and metropolitan areas a practitioner is likely to have patients from a wide variety of religious backgrounds. In many cases practitioners are working with people in the midst of life's biggest transitions, such as birth, death, or a major loss of bodily function. This is the very set of transitions that have been the province of religion since the beginnings of human culture. Add to this the fact that many practitioners are struggling with their own religious backgrounds and their own spiritual lives, particularly as they try to make sense of the suffering they place their hands on each day. We may say that, for the most part, our interviewees accept religious and spiritual beliefs and practices as part of a wide range of resources that can help the body heal. The fascination comes in watching how they work to manifest this in clinics, offices, hospitals, and field settings.[1]

ACKNOWLEDGING AND ASSIGNING MEANING

Medical culture, especially in a large medical center, both sees and presents itself to the culture at large as a culture of science. Often this culture of science is assumed to hold authority over religious traditions and communities. Furthermore, discussions of patient autonomy and the inequalities of power inherent in caregiver–patient relations provide important cautions for caregivers interested in offering or sharing religious and spiritual beliefs and practices with patients. In addition, there is the fundamental constitutional principle of freedom of religion in the United States. To put it baldly, coercion in the area of religion is not likely to be healing and is unlikely to be tolerated; it is unethical; and in most cases it is almost certainly illegal.

How, then, do our practitioners work with their patients through this set of entanglements? We begin with a psychiatrist's relatively straightforward and clinical diagnosis and assessment of resources:

> The spiritual is part of the issue, too. I will ask questions about belief systems. Since you became ill, have you prayed more? Since you became ill, have you thought differently? Have you become angry at He who represented the spiritual presence in your life? If I hear, for example, that a highly spiritual individual has become angry or cynical, or has basically given up on the Lord or his maker or that which would be theoretically a comfort to him, I will try to bring that person back into that fold. Which may not be my fold, but I don't care. I'm trying to bring him back into his. I want him to reconnect with his spiritual side, much as I would want him to reconnect with other aspects of his life which have been helpful in the past.

The critical matter here is, "Has there been a change?" What role did religious life and community have in this individual's life in the past? How can those potential resources be re-engaged? Another physician addresses directly issues of trust and power that run alongside any conversation between practitioner and patient about religion. Note in particular the stress on the importance of the opening query:

> I think that my obligation, like in any other domain of their life, is to create a trusting environment, where the patient is open to discussing religious things. I may even need to prod them a little bit, by asking a general question—something like, "Do you have a strong faith?" I think the thing that you have to be very careful about in this unequal power relationship is somehow abusing that power. I come from a Christian background, and that means that I've got to be careful that I don't, somehow, imply that that's the only way to believe. Or that my approval of them is going to be based on their agreeing with me on matters of religion.

Matters of "coercion" in these domains can be very subtle. Implicitly eliciting—or even subconsciously needing—the agreement of a patient about religious matters is a breach of trust. This matter of "not wanting to disappoint the doctor" is, in most settings, far more likely to be the intrusion on the patients' religious freedom than overt evangelizing.

> My credo is that with matters of faith and patients, it's certainly permissible and good to follow, but you should never lead. You can't be the one driving the ship. Now, you open that door and they walk through it, they want to talk about it, great. You open that door and they're noncommittal, then move on to something else. That's not a domain they want to go to, and you should not push that issue on them. Because that can abuse the power, the relationship, if you push that on them.

In this case there is a willingness to engage in a conversation with a patient on the basis of the patient's invitation, a conversation informed by the practitioner's own religious commitments. This moves beyond diagnosis and assessment and into a place of accompanying the patient, of exploring with him or her.

A particularly sensitive and thorough account of this "back-and-forth" between caregiver and patient in the domain of spirituality comes from a neonatologist.

> I: Do you have a working definition of healing from your own experiences dealing with patients and families?
>
> P: I suppose I would fall back on the old term "holistic" or "holism." Looking at healing as being representative of physical, emotional, spiritual aspects. It's a sense of being complete or whole as it is . . . I would even say it might be peace. A sense of peace about who I am, what my condition is, and what that condition means. I'm talking about meaning in a grander sense. What a person wants to hear is, "This means my child is going to be able to do x, y, or z." Go to college, play sports, run and jump, not have learning disabilities, and so on. So the meaning of the condition has to be conveyed in that larger sense, whether that's a spiritual or religious framework, secular humanist, or any approach, whether or not the parents confirm a spiritual dimension and are open about that. We may address it, and if they're not open about that, then it's generally not attended to.

There is the initial statement of the multiple layers of healing that we are familiar with. And then there is the recognition that questions of ultimate goals and purposes of life will inevitably arise, along with ones about the openness of the future, the power of the past over the future, and the suffering of the child and the parents in present time. And yet, even so, there is that fundamental caution about intruding.

But this caution is immediately followed by an explanation of what would drive the practitioner to insist on certain kinds of conversation in a way that, in other circumstances, might well be considered inappropriate.

If we're in dire straits and a child, if the child is gravely ill and we may not see him survive, then the meaning issue takes on a greater significance. We may be discussing issues of therapeutic trials or limits or withdrawal of life support or certain highly risky interventions. The meaning issue then takes more of our attention. And whether, again, it's spiritual dimensions or otherwise, there's more language addressing that, there's more time addressing that.

The relatively neutral and noncommittal terms like "meaning issue" and "attention" serve to hold an open space for a variety of responses from the patient's parents, and to guide the caregivers' attention. There is an enormous schooling in sensitivity that is in evidence here. But, almost in the same breath, another situation requiring an otherwise unacceptable level of intervention is described:

There have been occasions where I see that the assignment of meaning is unhealthy and actually not serving a good for the parents. "This has been a test from God." Or, "This was due to the fact that I did or didn't eat, drink, smoke, expose myself to, or take certain action during pregnancy." There's a lot of this guilt that is part of adverse pregnancy outcomes that women bear. And I feel the responsibility as a healing physician to convey reassurance that, "No, you need to disregard that. That guilt is inappropriate." We need to allay these anxieties. Sometimes that becomes very important. Early on in a hospital course, or if the course is on a grave illness and potential death, then, "No, it's not your fault." That's what I mean by attending to inappropriate assignment of meaning. I think it's my responsibility to do that.

The prospect arises here of the practitioner standing in opposition to a patient's religious belief or religious community. But the practitioner is very clear where her responsibility as a healing professional lies.

And then there is the fact that these conversations, and such interventions, are likely to take place in the course of a prolonged series of interactions between doctor and patient.

> If I've seen and managed a baby and a family for a number of weeks and I'm touching base with them, there's usually a handshake for mom and dad. And if they express concern, I may say, "We've been through this before. The information is here." Or, "We're going to learn this with this test. Bear with us and continue to keep your faith." I often say this to parents and even healthcare team members. "Keep your fingers crossed and say your prayers, and everything is going to be okay." Whether you believe in good luck or fate or the gods . . . and I have some parents come back and say that it was important for me to say that. I don't say it intentionally. It's become sort of a habit.

It is as if the progression of interactions between the practitioner and the parents move inexorably towards "the meaning piece," the "spiritual dimensions." And, concomitantly, that it would be unnatural or inauthentic not to acknowledge that, not to pick it up in one way or another.

Sometimes parents make it quite clear from the beginning that they belong to a religious community or tradition.

> There have been circumstances where parents have conveyed explicitly a faith, "We're Muslims, and this is very important. Please do this." I abide by that. Or, "We're Jewish." "We're Christian." "We're Catholic." And acknowledging and attending to that—without personalizing that, or responding to that in a personal sense—is important for healing.

It is one thing to be prepared in principle and in conversation to deal with religious pluralism. But to have the staff and facilities, and the institutional willingness, to actually do what families from a broad range of religious communities ask is another. The emphasis on the instruction "without personalizing" is a first step towards preparing staff on levels for dealing with practices and behaviors that may be not just unfamiliar, but distressing or confusing or even offensive. And yet making room for a pluralistic population is essential:

> Because it's usually in that [religious] framework that people find or ascribe meaning of illness, or meaning of life circumstance, or meaning of death. I can acknowledge that and say, "I'm glad that you have that support." In fact, sometimes in dealing with critical illness, after conveying the condition of the child, I ask, "How is it that you go about making hard decisions in your family? Who's important for you to talk with? Family members? Friends? People in a faith community? Is it a psychologist or therapist or counselor? Who can we share this with that can help you in understanding and making these difficult decisions?" And I suppose doing that is part of being a healer, attending to who the parents are, and the meaning piece, once we've conveyed to them the condition of their child.

"Being a healer." In this context that means being open to the spiritual dimensions; it means being open to a wide variety of religious practices; and it means being open to the presence and contributions of family and community members.

THE RELIGIOUS AND SPIRITUAL ORIENTATION OF PRACTITIONERS

A significant proportion of our interviewees talked about their own religious traditions and practices, and how those commitments informed their clinical practice. For some it is about how such religion and spirituality shape medical practice. For others it is more about self-concept and self-care. For still others it is essential to any description of healing. And for many others, a mix of all three.

It is also worth noting that many of our clinicians have developed small rituals that are unobtrusive and yet formative. And it is likewise important to pay attention to how carefully our practitioners delineate the boundary separating what they do and believe from the patient's religious life, even when talking directly about the role of religion and spirituality in their own lives.

> I am a Christian, so I do say "God bless" when I see patients, and things like that. Nobody ever said that they were offended, although some people told me that they didn't believe in God. So I am still going to pray for them. I like people, and especially here in the South . . . that's just part of me.

For this practitioner, his sense of himself as a Christian comes into the way he greets people and parts from them. Two small words of ritual, and an intention to pray, flowing out of an interest in and a liking for people.

> But I think the key there is not to invade the patients' own belief, to let them have their own gods and their own cultures, and to honor those. I love to do a Hindu greeting, which I think tells it all: I respect the spirit within them. I'd do that sometimes and they look at me like, "What does that mean?"

Alongside the strict injunction not to interfere with patients' religious lives, there is an effort, in another small ritual, to acknowledge that "we are both religious people." This acknowledgment sets the doctor and the patient apart from, or makes them a small enclave within, the scientific culture and apparatus all around them.

Here a practitioner who also is Christian emphasizes the discipline involved in a life that follows the teachings of Jesus.

> I try to be a disciple of Jesus Christ. It's a hard discipline at times, and at other times it is not so hard. In terms of Biblical reading, I prefer the Gospels over Acts and the Letters. I do appreciate

the toughness of Jesus in dealing with certain kinds of people. But I tend to be a "social gospel" sort of person.

The clinician clarifies which part of Christian tradition is foundational for him and then clarifies how this informs his interactions with his patients.

In these conversations, I stay on the ethical side, not the religion side—although in this last few years I have been a little more open to religious conversation with patients. But there I suggest that exploring it might be good for them or helpful to them. My main objective is to show its importance in my own life.

There is, finally, the sense that a life lived by the discipline of the Gospels will show itself in actions, and that further words about belief or scripture are unnecessary.

It is important to recall that religious pluralism is a fact for any group of practitioners as well. This is often highlighted more dramatically in conversation with complementary or alternative medicine practitioners, because their traditions of diagnosis and treatment often do not assume the divide between religion and science that lies at the foundation of modern Western allopathic medicine.

I: Can you say more about this healing power that resides in the body that you're trying to release as you release bodily tension?

P: In chiropractic philosophy they talk about innate healing potential. "Innate intelligence" is the term they utilize. It's this global intelligence that created the planet.... You may want to think about it as God or whatever your own personal philosophy allows. Obviously, something with a very vast amount of intelligence participated in creating nature and the planets. It just couldn't have been totally haphazard. So what we try to do is to bring that concept down into the individual body and show that there is some of that innate intelligence that resides within each individual body.

Each body contains a spark of the divine intelligence. This is a common belief throughout the world's religious traditions. Here we see this conviction shaping an entire system of medicine. And yet there is no need to convert the patient. Much room is given for individual interpretation of the basic principle that the body has innate powers to heal itself.

Virtually the only theological discussion in the transcripts, and certainly the longest, came in an interview with a family practitioner. What is intriguing here is how he understands himself as a Christian, and not as an evangelist. This entails, once more, a specification of just which aspect of this tradition informs his life.

The need some of our interviewees felt to make these kinds of distinctions points to an often-unrecognized dimension of religious pluralism that we would do well to underscore here. There are, within all of the world's major religions, a quite wide variety of traditions, beliefs, and practices. This "pluralism" is often not well understood by the adherents of one form of religious practice as they think about other traditions. It may be helpful to keep these complexities in mind when reading the following explication.

I have done some mission work before, worked in a mission hospital. I have a strong motivation in my Christian faith to do lots of things. But I also feel it's important that, within the context of my practice, I'm not an evangelist. I am a Calvinist. Basically, Calvin says that God is responsible for everything that is good in our life. Even our ability to choose Him comes from God. It doesn't come from us. So I don't feel responsible for anyone else's faith. That is God's work. And if He's working on someone, or if He's revealing Himself to someone, that is not my responsibility. Thank goodness for them, and for me!

In turn, however, the physician is called to do another kind of work, and to be receptive to God's assistance as he does it.

But I also feel like I am this instrument of His work in this world. And if I believe that He has something good to offer, I should be open to that. There are things I do as often as I can. If I have a complex patient that I am going to see, I just say this quick prayer: "I don't have the insight to human nature like You do. Just help me find a key for what it is they need. Help me understand them well enough and love them well enough that I can understand what it is that they really need."

Once again, a very small ritual practice, this time quite private, involving neither the patient nor other caregivers, yet strongly informing the medical practice.

Part of it is spiritual, and part of it is also just the preparation of my own mind. So that I don't walk into a room with a need for a ready answer or with a sense of urgency, so that I don't rush the patient through the visit. When I do that prayer, I find that I am much more open to things that I wouldn't have been open to otherwise.

By removing totally any direct responsibility the doctor might be understood to have for the faith of his patients, and by opening himself to God's assistance, this practitioner finds himself able to see and to receive his patients more clearly and more fully.

A very different approach that can allow a person with one religious practice to make room for others with different practices is the common path of modeling oneself on a teacher, a sacred being, or an exemplary woman or man.

I ask myself from time to time, "Who are my ideals?" And I've always come back to three: Jesus, Gandhi, and Schweitzer. Those are three people that have meant a great deal to me. And the thing that, as I think of them, that they shared so prominently, is that they lived it. They lived it and then died it. The feeling that somebody who's willing to both live and die in accord with what

he believes: that's big-time stuff to me. And those three people
have somehow etched themselves on my cortex.

They live it, and they die it. They act, and act rightly, without
regard to unfavorable consequences. These three figures, drawn
from different times and cultures, are offered here in what might be
called a "generically religious" way. Anyone could seek to emulate
these three people, no matter what their religious background
or commitment might be. We may think of this practice as a manifes-
tation of religion and spirituality focused on action.

ENGAGING PATIENTS IN THE RELIGIOUS AND SPIRITUAL DIMENSION

While most of our interviewees showed awareness of religious pluralism and sensitivity to the problems that present in a clinical setting,
several practitioners talked more explicitly about their process of
handling differences between their own religious and spiritual practices and beliefs, and those of their patients. One practitioner
reported,

> At times I've tried brief entries into prayer with people, explicit
> prayer. And I'm not very good at words or prayers, so I gave that
> up. But there is an implicit sense of who a person is, what it
> means to be a self, and what the experience of that self is. And of
> how there's a holding on to that identity, and a respect for that
> holding on, because I do it myself. And a respect for other peo-
> ple's holdings on, whatever that may be.

There is the initial effort to engage his patients' own religious
practice and the recognition of failure. And then the stepping back
from that into a general or universal appreciation of the spiritual
life of each person—the "holding on," in a positive sense, to all that

constitutes one as a human being. This appreciation is not hindered but rather nourished by his own spiritual life.

> My own [spiritual] practice, in its highest sense, gives me a respect for how other people struggle, how we all struggle. And so I think that I do strive explicitly in myself to express that understanding, in relationship with people when they come to see me because they're hurting, for whatever reason.

His own practice offers a perspective on pain and suffering that shapes how he receives his patients. And this, even as he often sees how far his own religious life is from that of many of his patients.

> P: People say things to me like, "You know, God is working through me." Or, "I got better because the church family prayed for me." I have a mixed reaction to that because I don't share that fundamentalist view of God or a strict Bible interpretation. But I utterly respect the way that belief works in someone's life. And that belief needs support and respect. I struggle for ways to acknowledge that in people, without ignoring my own truth. It's a pretty common circumstance.
>
> I: I expect it would be.
>
> P: Again, I'm thinking about my own personal issues mixed into that. I was raised Jewish; I practice Buddhism. I don't share those things with people a lot.

A central puzzle for practitioners is highlighted here. The complexity of a practitioner's own spiritual and religious development can sometimes become evident and perhaps more vivid through his or her encounters with the religious or spiritual dimension of patients' lives. The resulting puzzle can be expressed as a question: How can clinicians draw upon their own spiritual traditions to promote healing in their patients when these traditions are not only distinct from, but in some cases in direct disagreement with, the beliefs and practices of their patients?

One acupuncturist's approach sheds light on this puzzle:

> Chinese spirituality is not in the best interest of many patients. I sometimes tell people to "go home and pray about it" to see if this kind of treatment is the right thing for them. I'm always looking for the spiritual grounding of the patient and for how to link that up with their health care. I was raised by "foot-washing Baptists." I've got deep respect for and understanding of those folks.

Her own biography grounds this clinician's awareness that the religious beliefs and practices underlying the form of Chinese medicine practiced in her clinic may make some therapies offered unhelpful or even damaging for some of her patients. And this damage may be present even though there is no effort to "convert" the patient from being a "foot-washing Baptist" to a Taoist adept. This potential conflict resolves itself for this practitioner on another level:

> The deeper I go into my own path, the less need I have for others to share that path—the easier it is to accept others where they are.

By schooling herself in a tradition likely to be quite foreign to that of the vast majority of her patients, this doctor finds herself more and more able to make room for people's varied spiritual paths.

Yet there can be complications for the practitioner, and thus also for the patient, that arise as the caregiver attempts to make room for the patient's religious life. In these cases, the patient's religious life can be intrusive.

> P: One issue that is tough for people—it's tough for me, sometimes—is what to do, how to handle certain kinds of spiritual issues, or certain kinds of faith stuff that comes up in the nature of the encounter.
> I: For example?

P: For example, requests to pray for patients, or to pray with patients. It can get complicated for me, because I rarely share the same faith belief as patients around here. How do you respond to that in a way that doesn't hurt the relationship, but doesn't have you doing anything that's not sincere? I think that ends up actually, for a number of people, being a reason not to go there with some of this stuff. Because you're afraid it might go further than you meant it to go, and then you don't know how to extricate yourself.

There is the relatively simple matter of not sharing the same religion, but then there are the further, more subtle issues of trust and authenticity. One wants to be present, but without compromising one's own integrity, or that of the relationship with the patient.

And finally there are those cases where the practitioner sees a patient's religious stance hindering their healing.

I've seen many, many patients over time whose belief systems got in the way of their healing process. Because many times they are taught not to allow anything in that isn't the Gospel, and what that does is interfere with the experience of healing. I have my opinions of what spirituality is, as other people do, of course. But I sure see times where I would walk out kind of shaking my head going, "I can help this person, if they could open up."

The phrase "open up" invites questions. Would "opening up" mean setting aside one's religious tradition for another? A conversion, in short. Or would it be a different way of carrying that tradition? Or would it mean being somehow "nonreligious"?

I believe that a lot of religious practices get in the way of opening up. But now, as I say this, I'm finding in my imagination a person with a very, very narrow concept from the Western medicine side who says, "What's he talking about? You Chinese doctors are the ones who are doing the religious practice here." But personally,

I just can't imagine you can do healing work without bringing Spirit in. Now, it doesn't necessarily have to mean that whoever comes in has to practice Taoism or Buddhism.

So over against the "narrow concept from the Western medicine side," this practitioner uses the word "Spirit" and claims that no healing happens without it. And he makes it clear that the traditions associated with Chinese medicine are not essential for one to "bring Spirit in." The key, once more, is openness:

But it does help if the mind is open, if there is receptivity. I don't think healing can work if we have a hardened being, and that's part of what this is about, is to soften it.

What can be done with "hardened being"? What's involved in "softening" up? It is just this kind of inquiry that leads many practitioners to emphasize a very broad conception of healing, one that includes a spiritual dimension. It is just this kind of inquiry that leads them to talk freely about those religious teachings, stances, and practices that open the wounded life to healing in its largest sense.

HEALING, CENTERING, WHOLENESS: "PEACE IN THEIR EYETEETH"

When asked to talk about healing, and how healing happens, almost all our practitioners acknowledged that healing is more than physical, more than repair or cure of the body. What this "more than physical," "more than curing" might be is depicted in a number of ways. One of the most common introduces "holistic" and "wholeness" into the discussion.

The holistic sense of healing really has so much to do with finding yourself in time and space and being satisfied. Locating yourself. The process of locating yourself in respect to the world around you and the people around you. Many people are lost in time and space, and so I think healing has to do with centering yourself.

Finding one's place in the cosmos—in place and time, and in community. Is there a more fundamental question addressed by religious traditions? And what does the process of "locating oneself" involve? First, we are given the word "centering," which brings to mind various meditation techniques from Eastern traditions, and the Christian process of "centering prayer."

> I: Can you think of instances in which you think your patients have achieved something like this? Where you want to say that this is a person—maybe it turned out really well, in terms of their health status, or maybe it didn't—but that they had a healing experience?
> P: Yeah, I think a lot of times it had to do with that acceptance . . . once they found where they were, or accepting whatever location where they found themselves in. Finding yourself and accepting your location for what it is, and being satisfied with it.

Part of "not being healed," of being lost in space and time, of being ill, would then be a refusal of the place where you know you are. And the movement to healing would come with a clearer view of where you are, and a deeper acceptance of that. Which could, in turn, be a definition of "being centered."

Another approach to a broader conception of healing emphasizes life outcomes and enduring identity.

> First of all it is, I think, the ultimate outcome in the person's life. I think that on a psychological level, that it's constantly reliving an area of dissonance, until the piano is tuned, until there's healing—we're working towards that, though it may never happen.

Initially, two levels are distinguished. That of "the ultimate outcome in the person's life," of their degree of fulfillment or completion, in the broadest and most nuanced sense. And then the psychological level, where we are understood as "constantly working things out."

> Patients will ask me about healing and want to be healed, and this comes up where faith, or the idea of faith, has to do with healing. There's a lot of linkage there, and they may feel like a failure with their faith because their body isn't being healed. To me, that's almost the biggest emergency.

"The biggest emergency" is a striking phrase. And especially so, since it comes not from a chaplain or religious teacher, a psychologist or psychiatrist, but from a physician who works daily with cancer patients.

> I learned this phraseology as a fellow, when I walked into a woman's room who had colon cancer. In her forties, herself a hospice chaplain. She would start each encounter saying, "My faith will make me whole, and I'm going to be healed of this. I'm already healed of this." And then her move to anger, this unbelievable anger that comes through people when they're angry at God and they don't feel safe feeling that. All I knew to say as I sat with her was, "There's a part of you that the cancer will never be able to touch." Just to say that, and identify or separate out who she is from what's happening to her physical body.

There is an essential part of you that is not harmed by the deterioration of the body. There is a wholeness that encompasses not only the body as it is stricken by cancer, but death as well.

> And I went on to say to her that healing can look like different things, and you may not die healed, but you can die whole. You can die a whole person. And that seemed to give her peace. So

I think for a person to be healed—I think of little circles. That's one reason why I wear these bracelets, and I play with them a lot, is I think of overlapping circles of influence. And that, for a person to have peace in their eyeteeth, whatever that means to them—that is a form of being healed.

"Peace in their eyeteeth." Reaching as deep a peace as is possible: this is what it is to be healed.

The question of identity, of who and what one really is, comes to the forefront as well in the following account from an acupuncturist.

In Chinese medicine, for serious conditions, there's always some aspect of phlegm. The spleen system manufactures phlegm; the lung system can store phlegm. The kidneys, or the kidney system, can transport phlegm. And the heart system can evaporate phlegm. So in Chinese medicine if there is a miracle according to Western medicine, it's because there's a heart aspect involved.

The first step is that Chinese medicine has an explanation, within its own understanding of physiology, for what in Western medicine would be found "inexplicable" and thought of as a "miracle," and perhaps a "religious miracle." In Chinese medicine, the heart is the "miracle."

It's like, on some spiritual level, the heart opens or sees or accepts some part of that individual, and the phlegm evaporates, and the condition goes away.

Acceptance of one's self, embracing those parts of one's self that have been pushed away, for whatever reason, is the opening of the heart—which may be otherwise described as forgiveness, or as compassion. These themes will recur.

In Chinese medicine, there's always some aspect of daily life that creates, or helps to create, that condition. And yes, you may have been born with a propensity for that to develop. But based on your lifestyle, it develops. In Chinese medicine, that shift in the energetic system of the heart that allows the evaporation of that phlegm and the miracle to occur, is religious or spiritual in the sense that a human being has some spiritual shift in who they are.

The heart shift is a religious or spiritual shift. Such a shift involves changes in daily life that address both the symptoms and the inherited tendencies. But the first movement is the opening of the heart.

This analogy just occurred to me—conversion : healing. Conversion to a faith, and healing. You do it one person at a time. It's very individual. It's not, typically, group work. People have to find their own way to faith, to belief. And people have to find their own way to healing. I'll have to play with that analogy a little bit more. Maybe it works; maybe it doesn't.

What he is proposing is to be clearly distinguished from the idea that conversion to any particular religion brings about or is necessary for healing. Rather, he is suggesting that true and deep healing involves the total transformation of a life, on the order of that transformation one associates with religious conversion.

As expected, many practitioners struggle with dilemmas generated by their commitments to "hard science" and their own spiritual lives. But some also struggle with dilemmas created by their commitment to the "hard science" they see as the basis of their clinical work, especially as they are confronted with phenomena that "hard science" cannot account for.

P: I fluctuate from being a very . . . not spiritual, but a person who believes that there is another reality that we don't have access to. I fluctuate between that and being a hard scientist. And then I look at the babies, and I think, "Where is this stuff about healing fitting for the babies?" I have a well-established sense of how it works with the families and the different levels of healing that happen. But there's a part of me that would really like to know how could we apply this to the babies. Because the placebo effect doesn't work with babies. They don't have the ability to believe in their treatments.

I: Perhaps a level of awareness with the babies, even though it wouldn't fit under expectancy of improvement? Something there that is received?

P: It just seems that, when you have people who have this rosy optimism, that their babies do better than the ones who are scared of everything. There's something going on. The babies do better. I don't know whether it's us, whether it's the baby. . . . So that's my big question: how does it fit with the babies?

We know there are beneficial aspects of positive human relationships. Positive regard and deep connection clearly support health and healing. But how? "How does it fit with the babies?" If there is a fundamental point about healing that everyone agrees on, it is that healing is a mystery.

We can give nutrition; we can support with the ventilator or dialysis or vasoactive agents. We can support bodily functions. But healing comes from down deep inside, from powers that we don't really control. I use that language with families, to help them understand that all we can do as humans is support functions that we know are necessary for life. But we can't force healing to happen. Those are powers beyond ours.

Practitioners know they do not do the healing themselves. But if those powers are beyond ours, how then do we approach them?

RELIGIOUS RITUAL AND THE PROCESS OF HEALING

Religious teachers and communities have, virtually always and everywhere, understood ritual to have healing power. In most traditions, these rituals are both supported by, and supportive of, the common themes and teachings we are examining in this chapter: humility, for-giveness, compassion, surrender, gratitude. While recognizing clearly the need to make room for a wide range of religious practices, a number of our practitioners talked specifically about two major sets of religious ritual as important for achieving healing: prayer and meditation.

Prayer and meditation are two of humanity's most fundamental ritual practices. Both are found in the civilizational religions of the East and the West. Even so, it would still be fair to say that prayer is foundational practice in the West, as meditation is in the East. Many of our practitioners spoke about these rituals and the importance each can have in a healing process. And a few spoke at length, and quite knowledgeably, about them. Sometimes this conversation moved around praying with patients, or teaching meditation to patients. At other times, it moved around the importance of prayer and/or meditation in the practitioner's own life and healing work. Thinking again of the "pragmatics" of religion, one may approach these rituals as activities that help remove blockages or remake con-nections in the life, the world, and the body of the patient. And we know by now from listening to our practitioners that medical prac-tice itself, broadly considered, may be understood as just that: remov-ing blockages and remaking connections so that the powers of healing that reside in the body can successfully do their work. Picked up in this way, religious ritual may be understood as complementing and supporting medical therapies and interventions.

Prayer

The topic of prayer is approached with great care by our caregivers. This is, in part, out of respect for the practice itself. But it is also due to the tremendous amount of attention intercessory prayer for heal-ing has received in national and local media, in religious communities, and in certain portions of the scientific community. Commonly overlooked here is the fact that there are many forms of prayer and many different prayer practices. But it is not surprising that interces-sory prayer—prayer for the healing of a specific person or group of people in a specific time and place—dominates the vast majority of discussions of religious ritual and healing. A few of our practitioners did mention contemplative prayer practices. But overall the general tendency to concentrate on intercessory or petitionary prayer held true for our interviewees as well.

We begin with a practitioner who talks about how he engages the prayer practice of patients who do not share his religious beliefs in order to facilitate their healing:

> In terms of spiritual involvement with healing . . . we live in an interesting community. Fundamentalist Christians are a big contingent. So when somebody with beliefs like that presents in my office and they make me aware of the fact that they prayed to be healed, I definitely try to encourage that. Prayers are powerful, and I always tell them, "If that's part of your life, let's definitely incorporate that into your healing process." And then I'll try to facilitate that with them. I try also talking a little bit of philosophy with them, suggesting that sometimes we can think that everybody has within their own body a part of God, a part that resides within their own body. If we can just allow that expression to happen a little more, unexpected and amazing things can happen.

A place is immediately made for the role of prayer in healing, alongside the healing modalities this practitioner offers. But in addition, there is a willingness to engage, to a limited degree, in a theological or philosophical conversation with the patient, which is itself also aimed at releasing the body's healing power.

The most extended discussion of intercessory prayer in our interviews is an exploration by a Christian practitioner who prays with and for his patients with great regularity, and has attended carefully to the interrelationship of his faith and his medical practice for decades. He begins his account by describing how he talks with his patients about their life stories:

> I found out early on that being able to listen to their life story connected me better with that child and that family, and then we

had a relationship. So, to begin with, and this is truthful strictly again based on my own perceptions of my faith, you connected to people through their life stories. We all have a story, and that story came from our Creator. If we can be sensitive to other people's stories, then we've got something going. I've always really enjoyed knowing where people were born, what their jobs were, where they lived, how many children they had. What did they enjoy in terms of going to movies, or what books to read— just the general stuff talking. And that then led to much more trust, and once trust is there you could have a sense of how to really effect a healing situation.

In this case, the practitioner gives emphasis to the life story based on (1) a theological understanding of that story; (2) his experience of the therapeutic value of connecting with his patients and their families through shared stories; and (3) his enjoyment of the telling and the listening. Frequently, this process of listening and sharing provides an opening:

I found that empathy could be acted out, once I identified that people were involved with a faith journey themselves, then empathy could be connected with prayer. Oftentimes, simply praying with the patient. And to me, praying with the patient . . . one way was, "God, will you do something here?" and then you touch a patient in a particular place. But most often I think it was a way of simply saying, "Hey, we agree to be concerned about this thing together."

Again, the emphasis on the human connection, like the emphasis on story, is important here. The role of empathy is highlighted: "We agree to be concerned about this thing together." This is the grounding of these prayers, rather than a shared set of doctrines, or some common understanding of God's agency. In certain situations, however, much more intimate rituals, rooted in very definite beliefs about God, healing and prayer, were conducted.

There is a woman who was head nurse of the children's ward at _____ Hospital who was diagnosed with MS. One of my colleagues and I prayed for her and anointed her with oil. And she swears to this day that she has never had another symptom. She swears that she was totally cured. All I do is simply accept what she said. I don't try to make anything out of it. You can come back and say, "Maybe that was not the correct diagnosis after all." I'm not going to argue with that.

There is the willingness to pray for healing, and the comfort and readiness to perform the ritual of anointing the patient with oil to bring about healing. And there is no effort to explain, no inclination to answer an objection or refute an alternative account. What was done was done and stands on its own as an act whose intent was healing. The moment of prayer, as it is recounted, is a moment of obedience and fidelity—and that is as far as the person praying can go.

I: I'm wondering if you can say a little bit more about the prayers that you have with patients and families. I'm sure you know that there's this effort now among several groups to look at the question of "Does petitionary prayer or intercessory prayer work?" With double-blind studies and groups of people praying for different kind of patients at a distance.

P: I have always prayed for the patient's condition and that God's power would alleviate that condition. I have always prayed for improvement, for healing. But I have never been dismayed. Once the prayer is done, I don't have any ownership of it. In other words, I think that when we're trying to look at validation and the double-blind studies, that's good and well. But then we're trying to institutionalize something that, from the beginning of the human race, has been part of our psyche/soul connection to the Creator. I feel like it's a sacrosanct condition that ought to be left alone.

Looking to prove the effectiveness of prayer, like having an attachment to outcomes of prayer, is to misunderstand the nature of prayer itself. No matter what the outcome, he says, "I have never been dismayed." Further, the empirical studies are presented as efforts to "institutionalize" a relationship that is a "sacrosanct condition that ought to be left alone." As religious teachers in a variety of traditions and communities have emphasized for millennia, prayer is not a matter of cause and effect.

There is another group of practitioners who, while comfortable participating in prayer initiated by the patient or a member of the patient's family or religious community, nevertheless prefer, as the interviewee below explains, to avoid wearing the religion "hat" while wearing the clinician "hat."

> I've never been comfortable with that—wearing the religious hat along with my doctor hat. If someone asks me to, I will. In such situations, I always try to participate, if their pastor is there or they're having prayer. I want to be part of that. I want to stand in the circle if they're holding hands and hold hands. I want to show respect for their beliefs and their faith and their hopes and their dreams and all the needs that they have. And you know, when you talk about healing, there are emotional and spiritual and physical and social dimensions always. It's multidimensional.

The participation rests on this practitioner's own religious convictions, and on his understanding of the complex nature of healing.

There are, however, times when practitioners who are attempting to make room for a patient's prayer life find themselves quite uncomfortable with the direction taken by the patient.

> A colleague of mine was making rounds on general medicine at the VA. She went into this patient's room with the usual twenty people. She does the visit, and at the end she asks, "Anything else we can do for you, Mr. Jones?" And he says, "I want you to pray with me." So she's suddenly on the spot, because she's got ten ducklings she's responsible for, and she herself is not a

113

particularly religious person. But she says, "Okay. That's fine," when she really didn't know what to think.

The discomfort here points to myriad differences between medical culture and religious culture. It highlights differences between religious backgrounds and attitudes about religion and ritual. And, in an additional turn, it underscores class differences as well:

So he grabbed her hand and another person's, and suddenly they become this little prayer circle. You know, residents and students and the pharmacist and whoever else. He then looks up at her and says, "Go ahead and start." And now she's getting really uncomfortable, but she goes, "Mr. Jones, why don't you go ahead and pray?" And so he starts saying, "Lord, please help me. Please pray for all these people," and he's getting into it, getting more and more animated, getting louder and louder. And, working himself up into a Pentecostal-type frenzy, he calls out, "Take the spirit! Take the spirit, someone! Take the spirit!" And he clearly wanted somebody else to pick up the prayer.

Part of what is at stake here is what we may call a matter of competence. The religious domain has, if you will, its own set of skills and knowledge, of crises and interventions. And, of course, there is no reason to expect a healthcare practitioner to have these competencies. What begins as discomfort becomes now a question of integrity and recognition of limits, for the clinician and the patient.

At this point, my colleague realizes she can't go on with this, and so she breaks in and says, "We all have respect for you and for your religion, Mr. Jones, but we can't go any farther at this point." And then she tries to stop it. At which point, he starts calling out, "Oh, Lord! They have science, but they do not have faith!" And so there's that fear—fear of something like that happening.

What we have here, in miniature, is a multifaceted conflict among several cultures that share too few assumptions to be able to come to mutual understanding and closure without an enormous amount of conversation, trust, and hard work—something not available on teaching rounds in most hospitals.

Our interviews suggest the yoking of medical practices with diverse rituals of prayer is a frequent occurrence and, for some combinations of clinician and patient, virtually inevitable. Even so, given the medical community's understanding of itself as scientific, and its widely shared understanding of science as antithetical to religion, this yoking is likely to remain unstable and discomforting for clinicians and patients, even as it is, for some, extraordinarily powerful, rewarding, and healing.

Meditation

Though without the deep cultural roots of prayer practices in the United States, and not nearly as widespread, meditation practices are rapidly coming to be recognized by caregivers of all kinds as healing resources. The nationwide prominence of Buddhist teachers and communities in Vipassana, Tibetan, and Zen schools has been a major factor in this "discovery" of these ancient practices. Especially important have been the highly visible conversations sponsored by the Dalai Lama between Tibetan Buddhist teachers and Western researchers on meditation, cognitive science, and healing. Likewise contributing to this trend is the now-pervasive recognition and acceptance of Chinese medicine, which includes a variety of meditation practices among its healing modalities, alongside acupuncture and herbal teas. In addition, well-known practitioners like Herbert Benson and Jon Kabat-Zinn have introduced a clinical approach to these rituals that has allowed them to be accepted in many medical arenas. Our interviewees have found ways to distill these teachings into practices that work in clinical settings.

Mindfulness techniques that are foundational for the Buddhist practices are quite commonly taught in the United States. These techniques are designed to help one be immediately aware of interconnections among bodily states, emotional states, and cognitive states—connections that mostly remain outside everyday consciousness.

The part of being mindful and my mindfulness work is very much connected to what's happening right now here and now. "I'm so angry at this patient. And it's all about me. What is it about me? Where am I going to put it?"

The fundamental assumption here is that one's response to other people is anchored in one's own needs and one's own history, regardless of the behavior of others. Mindfulness is an effort to examine those anchorages to provide freedom for a different kind of response.

"Can I love them where they are right now? Can I be fully open to them where they are?" Breathing and mindfulness are techniques to use with any healing relationship to continue to get back to who you're with, rather than stay with what you need. I teach this to supervisees, to nurses, to physicians. Take a breath when you're feeling a strong feeling. Breathe and take a minute. Ask yourself, "What's going on with me?" It's not about the other person. They're wherever they are.

Attention to breathing in such situations serves to disengage one's attention from other people and one's feelings about them, and to bring that attention back to oneself and one's own body. And because it is intrinsically relaxing, the intentional pausing for the breath also serves to introduce a degree of softness into highly charged encounters.

For some practitioners, it is regular mindfulness meditation that makes it possible for them to offer compassion consistently to their patients.

The energy of caregiving, of caring itself, remains a great mystery to me. It seems to me to spring from daily practice of meditation, contemplation, centering prayer, and deep listening. Being mindful each moment gives us the opportunity to help share in others' burdens, and offer compassion and understanding in the moment. And that to me is what caring is all about.

The full presence of the practitioner is required if patient encounters are to be healing. This is a dominant theme that emerged from our interviews. Meditation practices are here understood as ways of learning to be fully present in a single moment—present to oneself and to others. As such, these mindfulness rituals can be powerful healing resources for practitioners.

The most familiar forms of Chinese meditation in the United States are sequences of movements known as Tai Chi. Though associated in popular culture with the martial arts, many students of these ancient rituals would understand them to be a subset of a far larger set of mediation practices called Qigong. Qigong rituals include breathing techniques, Tai Chi movements, martial arts, and specific healing exercises. Though these elements of Qigong may be distinguished from one another for purposes of teaching and analysis, in practice they are typically fully integrated.

Qigong rituals are, in addition, correlated with the physiological systems that underlie Chinese medicine:

> There are specific Qigong exercises that you can do to address the different organ systems in the body. If you have liver cancer that's caused by an excessive liver condition, then there are sounds that you can make; and you make them loudly, because it's an excess condition. If it's a deficient condition, then you make the same sound; you just make it softly. There's a lot of research coming out of China right now about healing cancer with Qigong exercises. So one of the ideas behind the practice of Qigong and Tai Chi is to get centered and focused on the whole being. And to recognize in those movements that the body moves as a whole, very naturally, if you're paying attention.

There is a particular stress on the body's healing capacities and its innate wisdom in Chinese medicine. Qigong exercises are designed to move one out of ideas, thoughts, and emotions and back into various specific regions of the body where healing actually takes place.

And there's the simple Qigong. This is what you do. When you focus your mind here, you see the energy come in on the breath, you see it go out on the exhale. And what this does is start to bring energy to the first and second chakra area. But you can direct that energy anywhere. That's part of my training as a Qigong therapist. For example, you could take the points that were used in your acupuncture treatments and basically could go home and practice Qigong on those points and eliminate the need for acupuncture.

In Chinese medicine, then, a patient's "prescription" might include specific Qigong exercises focused on specific ailments and symptoms and their underlying causes.

And then there are in the interviews discussions of the "effects" of meditation, a subject as complex as the "effects" of prayer. Notice here a similar detachment from expectations and results to that we found in the discussion of prayer earlier.

P: People say, "Well, what do you get out of meditation?" Nothing; it is quiet. I have never had a vision of God coming down. When you first start doing that, you keep looking for some big deal. You don't get a big deal. What you get is the rhythm and the practice, and then you understand. You really begin to hear those around you a lot more. Your wife and your children— listening to them, because you thought you listened before.

I: Now you hear it.

P: Now you are beginning to understand that quiet is important for allowing their voices to be heard, not just yours.

"What you get" is a life shaped by being still, by centering. And that is a life that has more room in it for others, and for being truly present to others, than a life without meditation.

This process of making room within one's life can develop to the point that one has, so to speak, "room for the universe":

This sense of belonging to the universe, being part of the universe, is maybe the single most sustaining thing I do. And I literally do it while walking down to get the paper, or driving home. I do seek out quiet, and create quiet moments, but not on a schedule; not during yoga time or whatever, but anytime. You are part of the universe. So you just have to sort of say, "Oh, yeah. There you are, universe! You're great!" And you can do that even while in the middle of the street, if you're careful.

Part of the power of a daily ritual can be this day-in, day-out sense of belonging to the universe. And simply calling forth, in one's most ordinary moments, this awareness of belonging and being embraced by the whole of things can be profoundly healing.

HONORING THE MYSTERY

To be distinguished from our practitioners' discussions of traditional religious rituals are their explications of life-changing acts and admonitions formulated amidst their daily clinical practice, and largely derived from its realities. Our caregivers understand these acts and admonitions as various ways of honoring the mystery of healing. A quick listing of these would be similar to any listing of the fundamental teachings of the major religious traditions. In this section we will explore two of them, humility and vulnerability, and in the next section we will turn to forgiveness, surrender, and celebration.

A first step towards being a healer is recognition of the mystery of healing and that, paradoxically, it is not the healer who heals. Healing is not about the healer. Being a healer is about being in service to others—hence the emphasis on humility.

I cannot control one thing other than my own heart. I cannot control anything else. And then with that understanding, and with eagerness, to go out and do the work that we do in life. It doesn't have to be a doctor, could be anybody. Did God let that new person that I operated on die? But then the humility comes in, and that's when you really understand where you are to go in service of others. That's a message of all traditions. Seeing others and lifting them up when they're suffering—whether it be an emotional suffering, physical suffering. It is a beautiful thing.

Yet being present in the midst of life's most enormous passages, experiencing the range of power and emotion that goes with having such central roles in people's most transformative experiences, and having some part in outcomes of incalculable significance in people's lives make it hard to hold the stance of humility, to remember that it's "not about me."

> P: I think you always have to keep in mind, at least for me when I'm seeing folks is that it's not about me. You know, they just met me. They don't know anything about me.
>
> I: It's not personal.
>
> P: Yes, exactly. So don't take it personally. Your job is to be helping the patient, not just stroking your own ego. You're supposed to be helping them, whatever they want to do. You can demonstrate to them your compassion and your caring. Caring in that . . . I can get there earlier and stay there later and make sure everything is taken care of, because many of the patients aren't well cared for. You can, if you really care about what happens . . . some of the people are just so pitiful. I had this one boy who was the same age as my son with an 80 percent body burn, who amazingly survived. But you know, it just broke my heart. And so I stopped at the market on the way in to buy candy . . . things like that . . . if you do care about patients. And I think you can teach people. You can model caring.

Humility is an opening of the heart that allows fuller caring, and that allows one to hold, over time, the stance of service.

Related to humility, perhaps a precondition for it, is awareness of one's own vulnerability and, correspondingly, the vulnerability of all beings, all creatures. A Buddhist practitioner puts it this way:

> I think pain opens your heart. It can. It doesn't, necessarily. It can close your heart. But it carries the opportunity of opening

your heart and having compassion for others. One of the things I often hear is, "My brother always had back pain. I always put him down for it, always pooh-poohed it. Now I get it." Getting someone else's pain is a huge deal. So just compassion for other people, and awareness of your own body; a little bit more self-awareness.

This is the vulnerability that leads to compassion. I am vulnerable; others are vulnerable. I hurt; others hurt. It's not always about my pain. So compassion for my own suffering, and for the suffering of others.

The "wounded healer" is, of course, a central image and theme in Christian doctrine and practice.

When I was in the divinity school, I thought a lot about disability in terms of the Christian faith. About the power of believing in a Creator that would come down and share our disabilities, share our suffering, share our miseries. And to die disabled—stabbed in the side, hung up, in pain—to share that. And a whole healing process, too, which has to do with participating in people's disabilities or illnesses. Both as a physician, and as a human being.

The paradox here—suffering in order to heal, suffering with others in order to heal them—is a marker of the depth of the mystery of healing.

P: In a healing relationship—because these are vulnerable people—you'd better be vulnerable with them.

I: Right. So this notion of the healer who is also wounded.

P: Yes. Wounded. We're all wounded. And sharing our wounds with one another. It's kind of a relationship, a process.

I: This is an extraordinary and underappreciated motif about healers needing in a sense to be wounded. And to recognize their own woundedness in order to be . . . that empowers them. The ancients thought people who were defective in some ways . . . that was thought to be . . .

P: They couldn't hunt. They were crippled. But they got in touch with some other sort of spiritual power.

I: Right. So, they had special powers because of that, actually. Not in spite of it.

P: That's very good.

The wounded, the disabled, the "defective," the most vulnerable are understood in archaic and in civilizational religious traditions to be blessed with opportunities for approaching those unknown powers responsible for healing—opportunities often not available to those with lesser wounds, or those unaware of the degree of their woundedness.[2]

The directive is this: "You listen for the wound, and you let them know that you have wounds. You are not perfect."

FORGIVENESS, SURRENDER, AND CELEBRATION AS HEALING ACTS

Forgiveness may be thought of as embracing vulnerability, the wound, the lack of perfection, in others and in oneself. We are finding, in other words, that all these aspects of being a healing presence are interconnected, interrelated, and mutually supportive. We have already examined this formulation of the role of forgiveness in healing in Chapter 3. But it is worth looking at again in this context.

People who are not willing to accept forgiveness from those they have hurt, and those who are not willing to offer forgiveness to those who have hurt them, will live with the burden on their soul, with an aspect of bitterness and emotional constraint that they cannot get rid of, and that no amount of exercise, sleep, and diet is going to overcome. . . . We're going to hurt people at every turn in the road, and people are going to hurt us at every turn in the road. And if we choose to carry that burden, we will never be fully healthy.

What is especially clear in this presentation is the idea that a spiritual "flaw" or "deficit," being unforgiving, translates directly into illness. It has the ability to "trump" exercise, diet, sleep—all those things we think of as sustaining "good health."

When discussing forgiveness, many caregivers are careful to emphasize that forgiving oneself—and especially those parts of oneself that one finds most shameful, difficult, unappealing—is of critical importance for healing.

> One relationship that can be very healing is our relationship with ourselves. Can we relate to ourselves in a very different way, instead of being so angry with ourselves? Can we accept all of who we are? That's incredibly healing.

Forgiving makes possible that full interconnectedness that seems to invite the healing powers to come and work. And one way that happens, that those powers show themselves, is in the form of compassion.

Some of our practitioners speak of compassion. Others speak of love. There is hardly need here to speak at length of the role of love and compassion in traditions of healing and in the lives of healers. What is of particular interest at this juncture are the ways in which all these teachings can be woven into one another, almost to the point of becoming a single teaching. Here is one extraordinary formulation provided by a Jewish practitioner:

> Okay, it's not just his thing but you know, Jesus is love and that's it. And that's his description. He was the manifestation of love. Whatever spiritual leader you read, it all comes down to compassion. It comes down to communion. It comes down to love and being available. So how do you separate that from the healing process? You can't. He was the miracle healer, right? I mean, what was he doing? He was just giving away love free. If he ever existed, it doesn't make any difference. The idea is the same, you know. If you read any of the Indian guys, they're all talking the same stuff. You know, you've just got to be present for people. I'm a Jewish

guy quoting Jesus, right? He said unless you become as a child . . . and what is a child . . . a child is innocent, right? That's the whole [thing] . . . innocence. I can never understand the mental set of negativity. What is the point? If you have an option between yes and no, why would you pick no?

We find some practitioners who, when speaking of love, also speak of vulnerability, as if the two were yoked. One practitioner put it plainly and directly:

I have a heart and soul which I can offer them, which is the way of bringing them some love. Love is a tough word to talk about when you are talking about doctor and patient relationships. Do you love your patients? I think you have to. Some people don't want to say that they do, but I think in order to really get to the point of healing you have to love. You have to be compassionate, understanding, and willing to walk the wounded path with them.

And, as we found in Chapter 3, speaking of the role of love in healing often seems to be joined naturally to speaking of surrender. And notice also in the following account that surrender, rather than resulting in a diminishment of energy, actually leads to a heightened state that is understood as spiritual.

There are times I'm really in tune in myself, with my own surrender, healthy and vibrant. It's powerful to people. And when I have more energy at the end of the day than I when I started—that's when I set myself aside, when I surrender. Is that religious? I would not say that is religious, but I would say that's spiritual.

Surrender here has to do with a setting aside of self, with "getting out of the way" so that energies that surpass the ego's control can come into play. Next comes an exploration of surrender as it translates into relationship.

P: Do I have a spiritual relationship with people? I would say that relationship *per se* is spiritual. It is not intended to convey to the patient that it's spiritual, but I think it is.

I: That is a powerful image: "to surrender." And that it has to do with your surrender, not theirs. Or not some specific moment of surrender, but a stance?

P: I think it's ultimately what so-called love is. That word "love" is such a misused, abused, and misunderstood word. But I think, ultimately, that is what love is. It is to surrender.

Continuing to work the image of love and loving, this practitioner describes, in language few others would use, an experience many different practitioners allude to:

P: I've even thought about what people mean when they say they "make love." I say to myself, "How do you make love?" Making love is, if that's truly the case, when both people are totally surrendered. People are so surrendered—that's what it's like if you're making love.

I: Generative.

P: I think that actually happens in a nonsexual way, in the so-called doctor and patient relationship. I have felt that—as weird or as perverse as that may sound. But somehow physical touch, and just working with somebody . . . both parties are surrendered. There is a sense in which that love exists, and they don't know that. They may feel that, but it not like it's discussed—that would be too weird. But it is powerful and it happens.

Other interviewees talked in an almost mystical way of that moment in the consulting room when the walls fall away, and nothing is left but the concentrated world of patient and caregiver. Clearly, excellent personal boundaries are necessary if these states are not to transmute into unhealthy emotion and damaging behavior. But there is no avoiding this aspect of the healing encounter, this powerful dynamic of mutual surrender.

In the clinical arena, surrender of all kinds, including that of setting aside ego, finally rests on recognition of the limitations of what eventually can be done for a patient, of what human healers can do. This is one of the places that medical practice moves quite naturally into some kind of spiritual stance, some stance of release, some posture of letting go.

> So I will, early on, start talking about, "We're going to do everything that makes sense, everything that's humanly possible that makes sense here. But you have to understand that we're only human. There are certain things that we can do and certain things we cannot. But we're going to do everything we know how to do." So, at the end of this, when I'm saying, "We've done everything that was humanly possible, and it hasn't worked," they can recognize the distinction of what humans can and can't do. And so when we're stopping the human things, what's left is the spiritual component, which will be building throughout this, if there's a gradual decline.

Knowing that end-of-life situations lead inexorably to confronting the limits of human power, this practitioner works carefully to prepare for the conversation he knows is coming about letting go of control by bringing human interventions to an end.

Going further, some practitioners find in surrender the key to the deepest possible healing.

> If they can surrender—the deeper, deeper, deeper that they can surrender—the more available the work is. You can walk out of here with your shoulder pain gone, so that's pleasant, because then you can go on with your life. But if you are receptive, but deeper on an emotional level and spiritual level, and infinite levels . . . in the right moment, you could achieve consciousness, full consciousness. Any of us could. That's available to us at every moment, but we don't know how to surrender everything, to get there immediately.

Here some might speak of full integration; others might speak of the end of all alienation. Some might speak of accepting God's love; others might speak of union with the universe. The core of each, from this practitioner's perspective, is complete surrender. Surrender of all blockages and protection, of all ego-orientation and armor, of all need for control and understanding.

Corresponding to, and complementing, the "directives" we have already examined—humility, vulnerability, forgiveness, compassion, and surrender—is the presence of joy and gratitude and blessing. As one practitioner puts it,

> I've always said, "The final, common pathway to health is through joy." My coffee is good for me, because it is so full of joy. My chocolate that I eat every single day is good for me, because it is so full of joy. I think the final, common pathway is joy.

Another speaks of a sense of gratitude for life and the blessing that fully living can be.

> This living business, all of it, is mine, if I want it. It's as if great grace suddenly were to give us all the colors in the spectrum. It's as if possibilities that I didn't know existed were right there. This was no instantaneous, aha! kind of thing. But the outcome was this much more vibrant appreciation of being. So when I'm talking to my patients and trying to convey my side of the humanity equation, I'm probably saying, at least in part, "Let me share with you how exciting it seems to me that life could be."

Another practitioner talks about learning to recognize that one's patients are themselves gifts to the practitioner.

> One of the things that studying with our teacher has done is help me move to a place where I recognize more the holiness of each person. What he encourages us to do is to look at each patient as a light, and to reflect their light to them, so that they can see that

they're a light. And actually, in working with him, what I actually have also begun to recognize is that it's not just people who are holy. It's all things that are holy, and having a corresponding respect for all things.

Everything is holy, as mystics have taught for ages. And how extraordinarily fulfilling it can be when that sense of joyful appreciation permeates one's medical practice:

People are amazing, individuals are amazing, and humanity is amazing really. I think that is the inherent joy. What other profession can you walk into a room and have people tell you the most important thing in their life? There is no small talk. You just walk in and they say, "Let me talk about the thing that matters most in life." What a privilege.

[5]

PATIENT PERSPECTIVES: HEALING FROM THE OTHER SIDE OF THE BED RAIL

Directly the bed is called for, or, sunk deep among pillows in one chair, we raise our feet even an inch above the ground on another, we cease to be soldiers in the army of the upright; we become deserters.

—Virginia Woolf, *On Being Ill*

The practitioner seldom sees the onset of the condition that is brought to her. There is a crisis in the patient's world, understood as rooted in the body, by the time the patient gets to the clinician. The crisis may be major or minor in the eyes of the patient. But, either way, the patient fears a loss of a piece of her own world, or perhaps the loss of her whole world. And this fear, along with the changes, constitute the crisis: "I can't work." "I can't pick up my grandchildren." "I can't sleep." "My hand won't stop shaking." Something that used to be available to the patient no longer is. That is one definition of illness. And the hope of the patient, and her family, is typically that the world "as it was" be restored. That, in disease terminology, the premorbid state can be recovered.[1]

Nor does the practitioner see the initial treatments of the condition he is asked to address. By the time the patient gets to him, local resources have been exhausted. These resources most often include the patient's own self-care skills, the family's skills (parents, grand-parents, siblings, children) in caring for its own, and then, perhaps, the neighbor who is an EMT, or the old woman down the street who knows the herbs.[2] It is at the moment when all these reserves have failed that the patient, and often the family, decide to approach a clinician trained in one or another of the major medical systems available to them. The crisis may become overwhelming very quickly—a major accident or dramatic stroke where it is immediately clear that local resources will not be sufficient. Or it may come slowly: gradual loss of energy, of weight, of appetite. And it need not always be major: a cold, a cough that won't go away, a nagging back, pain in the knees. But however it happens, the patient seeks out the practitioner when an unwelcome change has occurred in his life-world, a change perceived as involving inextricably the patient's own body. And when the medical resources immediately at hand in the patient's world cannot successfully address the crisis.

In the chapters preceding this one, we have been attending to what practitioners say is most important to them in establishing healing relationships with patients. We want now to turn to that often underconsulted partner in healing, the patient. What do patients have to say about relationships with practitioners—and especially about what aspects of those relationships are healing? What do patients hope for, and what do they find, when they approach clinicians and ask for help in addressing crises in their world? Do the factors in establishing healing relationships identified by patients correlate in rough ways with what our extraordinary practitioners say they offer, or want to offer, when they are at their best?

The patient accounts and illness narratives selected for examination were chosen, in part, with the intention of covering a very wide range of "diseases," "diagnoses," "cases," "illnesses," "life-narratives." You will find in the pages that follow references primarily to accounts by people with severe, often fatal, conditions: cancer (spinal, breast, prostate, testicular, lymphatic), stroke, heart attack, paraplegia, mental illness (depression, bipolar disorder). The primary clinicians in almost all of these cases are physicians, drawn from a wide variety of specialties. But many types of caregivers—spouses, family members, and friends; therapists, nurses, and technicians—play enormously significant roles in these narratives of illness.

We would point out, however, that we refer, with a few exceptions, primarily to highly visible accounts of illness, mostly written by established authors (for instance, Virginia Woolf, Reynolds Price, Audre Lorde, Oliver Sachs, Norman Cousins, Kay Jamison, and William Styron). We have done this primarily because these works are readily accessible, and may already be familiar to, and serve as touchstones for, readers of this chapter. These patients join the less well-known but equally authoritative ones in offering observations about their own illnesses and healing, descriptions of their interactions with providers, and often striking insights into living in, through, or with a wound in their body-bound lives.

The problem, of course, in using written accounts, and a disproportionate number of well-known ones at that, is that what we have in hand is a skewed sampling of patients in the healthcare universe. Some gaps are glaringly obvious. Missing are the voices of the poor. Underrepresented are the voices of women and people of color. Making media more accessible to the missing will be an important step in researching and preserving illness narratives. And—a distinct yet related point—unaccounted for in the world of print are the vast populations for whom oral traditions are the primary method of preserving memories and engaging in reflection. The expanded use of the tools of ethnography and oral history and the resources of performance studies and playback theater in collecting and exploring illness narratives should be a priority for researchers and all others interested in relationships between practitioners and patients. Our task in this chapter, then, is to examine what our selected group of illness narratives has to teach us about healing relationships between patients and their practitioners. What we have found is corroboration of key points in our interviews with practitioners, but expressed with the immediacy and urgency that comes with, and is a significant part of, a major crisis in one's life.*

DISEASES AND ILLNESSES

> Talking to doctors always makes me conscious of what I am *not* supposed to say. Thus I am particularly silent when I have been given bad news. I know I am supposed to ask only about the disease, but what I feel is the illness.[3]

The encounter with the person chosen to be one's healthcare provider is one of the most fraught, overloaded, and potentially intense interactions human beings have with one another. You would have to look to family—to parents and children, to siblings with one another, and to spouses and partners—to find relationships as charged with spoken and unspoken hopes and fears, with conscious and unconscious needs and motives. And then there is the fear of the healer and the corresponding overinflation of the healer's importance. This makes for a complex dynamic involving the desire for a powerful healer, and the distrust of such power and its potential to harm those who are already vulnerable. And the more dire the situation, the more challenging all these dynamics become. This is so, and has apparently always been so, in every form of human culture. And it is into this matrix that the practitioner steps every time he or she opens an exam room door or steps up to the bedside in the hospital.

One's life is wounded. And one is expected to turn that life over to, most often in the American healthcare system a relative stranger

---

* A stylistic variation in this chapter should be noted at this point. When we are recounting highly charged interactions between patients and practitioners we will often use the "historical present," narrating past events in the present tense. This is true when we are speaking of the experiences of particular patients, and also when we are describing generic features of the patient-practitioner interaction. Our intention is to retain some of the immediacy and drama of these high-stake encounters. For the same reason, we also alternate between "he" and "she," and "him" and "her" in order to signal gender-neutral language, without interrupting the flow with the more cumbersome "he or she."

and say, in effect: "Help me recover what I've lost." Or: "Help me get back as much as possible of what I've lost." Or: "Keep me from losing this completely." One goes to a practitioner with a bodied wound, a "wounded world," vulnerable to begin with. And then, doubling that vulnerability, one says, by simply showing up: "I cannot fix myself. I need your help." Thus a doubled vulnerability, and a doubled fear: First: "Will you help *me*?" Second: "Can I be helped?"

In the ensuing interactions there is constant negotiation about how much knowledge or recognition of their world patients will be offered. But always there is the hope that the practitioner's knowledge and skill will resolve one's ruptured life by helping to heal one's illness. Which is to be distinguished from that grand and impossible hope that the clinician will fix the patient's entire world, will heal entire lives. Mostly, though, all hopes will remain unspoken. Most patients experienced in the ways of biomedical culture have learned the rules of appropriate speech. And those rules, for the most part, enjoin patient silence about the bulk of the realities of their own lived world. Arthur Frank puts it this way,

> The questions I want to ask about my life are not allowed, not speakable, not even thinkable. The gap between what I feel and what I feel allowed to say widens and deepens and swallows my voice.

The patient fights against the prevailing assumption that recognition is somehow too much to ask for, shows weakness, shows a need to be coddled.

> Physicians are generally polite about answering questions, but to ask a question one must already imagine the terms of an answer. My questions end up being phrased in disease terms, but what I really want to know is how to live with illness. . . . I do not want my questions answered; I want my experiences shared.[4]

As is widely known, too often in biomedicine just this sharing of experience does not occur. And this in spite of the fact that when we occupy the patient role—when we are the "designated patient"—we all hope at the very least that the existence of our world is acknowledged, as well as the frightening fracture in that world.[7]

As strategy of orientation for what follows, let us post now what might be considered the two outside poles of the very broad spectrum of patient hopes and expectations. We begin with Reynolds Price's description of his fundamental hope, which he sees as a minimal expectation, or even requirement:

> And surely a doctor should be expected to share—and to offer at all appropriate hours—the skills we expect of a teacher, a fireman, a priest, a cop, the neighborhood milkman or the dog-pound manager.
>
> Those are merely the skills of human sympathy, the skills for letting another creature know that his or her concern is honored and valued. . . . Such skills are not rare in the natural world.[5]

And for those doctors who choose not to offer this, Price proposes that this warning notice be posted on office door or lab coat: *"Expert technician. Expect no more. The quality of your life and death are your concern."*[6]

And then there is Anatole Broyard, who expresses the hope that his physician will engage his metaphysical self—his sense of aesthetics, of drama, of the need for a higher criticism.

> Now that I know I have cancer of the prostate, the lymph nodes, and part of my skeleton, what *do* I want in a doctor? I would say that I want one who is a close reader of illness and a good critic of medicine. . . . Also, I would like a doctor who is not only a talented physician, but a bit of a metaphysician, too. . . . There's a physical self who's ill, and there's a metaphysical self who's ill. When you die, your philosophy dies along with you. So I want a metaphysical man to keep me company. To get to my body, my doctor has to get to my character. He has to go through my soul. He doesn't only have to go through my anus. That's the backdoor to my personality.[7]

Somewhere in between lie Jill Taylor's 40 statements about what she needed for recovery from her stroke from her caregivers: physicians, therapists, and friends. Here is a representative sample:

- I am not stupid, I am wounded. Please respect me.
- Approach me with an open heart and slow your energy down. Take your time.
- Make eye contact with me. I am in here—come find me. Encourage me.
- Touch me appropriately and connect with me.
- Speak to me directly, not about me to others.
- Cheer me on. Expect me to recover completely, even if it takes twenty years![8]

Many patients, like Broyard, are hoping for a guide, and are fortunate if they can find a companion. All hope to avoid being traumatized; all hope to avoid being turned into a subhuman body, an inhuman creature with no feelings, dreams, or thoughts worthy of notice. Most are realistic enough to know that insults to their human being will occur. All hope for Price's basics. But this is now so unusual as to warrant special mention in almost every patient account reviewed for this chapter.

The practitioner of course feels the weight of such widely ranging expectations and typically meets them with no training—or no opportunity, given the biomedical system in which they work—to address such matters. Nor the inclination, in so many cases, given the selection and training processes so common in even the best medical schools across the country. These factors, combined with the considerable inherent risk of opening oneself to enormous suffering, generate correspondingly enormous fear in clinicians. And this fear is often managed by refusing to get involved in the illnesses of their patients.

Hence the practitioner one is most likely to see in the United States will be an allopathic physician who has undergone a regimen of biomedical training all too often focused on what may fairly be called a nonentity: a diseased body thought to be somehow separable from lives and worlds of the physician and of the patient. A body assumed to be approachable, and treatable, as a complex of unbalanced or unstable physiological dynamics by another such body.

This abstracted approach has the immediate disadvantage of cutting out two of the most important figures in healing: patients themselves and the primary caregivers in their lives. Without these two engaged, the clinician has almost no chance to succeed. But those both inhabit the patient's world that includes and is rooted in and sponsored by the patient's body. But a body approached physiologically reveals no evidence of "a patient," much less a caregiver. And thus no evidence of illness or of healing—only of disease and lack of disease. So much of patient narrative material is concerned, not unexpectedly, with how those two key players—the patient and the primary caregiver—are kept actively engaged in the process of healing their disrupted, mutual world. We will return to the role of the primary patient caregiver later in this chapter. For now we will focus on the fact that, in our accounts, practitioners are evaluated more often in terms of whether they help patients stay present and involved in their own healing process than any other matter. To be sure, the question of whether the clinician can do the technical work is critical: handle the procedures, select the right tests, prescribe the best medications. None of our patients, nor we ourselves, are saying that technical competence isn't critical; clearly it is. But in virtually a single voice, those providing our accounts say that the technical alone is insufficient.

After all, when we are patients, most of us want to be partners in our own healing. Partnership here we would understand minimally as a type of cooperative relationship, based on shared goals and assumptions. And if we find that we are not partners with our practitioner in the healing process, then *it is actually not our world being fixed*—but some isolated abstraction within a medical system of labels and interventions. An abstraction, furthermore, that one can only minimally identify with. Try as we might, most of us can't for very long think of ourselves as "the hip in 672," or "the lymphoma in 1014."

Acts of naming, even such shorthand identifications, so often taken as trivial or routine, are actually immensely important. Rooted in the diagnostic systems and practices of a given medical system, naming is one of the greatest healing powers the practitioner has. The practitioner gives a name to something you cannot name. And that naming brings it into your world where you can engage it. Unnamed, it lies outside your world and remains a threat to the whole world, not just a piece of it.

But the key point for the patient is: Does that naming done by the clinician actually name something in my world? How do I have confidence in how the naming was done? Confidence in the name itself? Or is it just a name being moved around out there that gets glued onto me?[9] If, as a patient, my sense is that the clinician has not "recognized" me as me by recognizing my world and the crisis *in that world* that brought me to him, then there's little reason to hope that the name he comes up with has anything to do with *my* life, with *my* illness. It may be a name within the medical system in which the clinician is trained. And the clinician may be very, very good at the naming game within that system. But the patient's not ungrounded fear is that that may well have nothing to do with naming a piece of her world. And without that confidence that the naming is about me and my world, the patient will be able to bring forth little confidence in the clinician. And without that, healing becomes steadily more unlikely.

The patient then brings two basic anxieties into the encounter with the physician. There is the anxiety about being seen. And the anxiety about whether the world in which they were living can be restored. The point we want to emphasize is that for the patient, the seeing, or being seen, or not being seen, comes first—a fact that many clinicians fail to realize. And why first? If the practitioner does not see my world, how do I know that it is my world that is being addressed by the practitioner, and not some sector of the medical world in which he lives? So often there is not congruity or even contact between the patient's world and the medical world. Medical system intervention can exacerbate the disruption of the world already in motion that brought patient to clinician in the first place.

Or the intervention can initiate some separate disruption entirely, which has the unfortunate "side effect" of making the healing, the curing, even the fixing of the first condition more difficult. And in both situations the patient's resources and those of his family now have to be diverted to deal with this additional rupture.

ENGAGING THE PERSON TO TREAT THE PATIENT

> I'm nervous. You're always nervous the first time (defensively); well I'm nervous every time. I imagine you, I don't know if your eyes will see me, or if you'll look beyond me as you find me lacking, wanting, not enough, not sufficient for my own story. At this point, it doesn't matter to me if you are a man or a woman—I just want you to be present with me; to touch me, to hear me, and to see me. I prepared for you; I rehearsed for you (charmingly).[10]

In first meetings, there can be anticipation of so many ways of not begin seen: Will I even be looked at? Will eyes engage with me? Or will they look beyond? Will seeing begin only then to have the eyes turn away, uninterested? Tessa Carr's performance journal gives a vivid sense of the degrees of vulnerability, and of intimacy, wrapped into an anticipated first appointment with a physician. "I prepared for you; I rehearsed for you."

We first present vignettes showing clearly that when patients are asking for recognition of their illness and their living worlds, they are not necessarily asking for huge amounts of time or a deep degree of emotional involvement. Indeed, the vast majority are not. What is wanted is what Carr is hoping for: "I just want you to be present with me; to touch me, to hear me, and to see me." This so often is a simple matter of gently placing a hand, a direct look in the eye. These are minimal skills, with measurable observables that can be altered with relatively simple training. Though there is, finally, something that is much more complex, which is developing a stance of attentiveness, or a bodily attunement to the enormity of body-rooted crises in the patient's world. Mastering attentiveness and attunement are life work, yes. But they are best begun with the simplest acts of recognition.

> Reynolds Price: "But the young presiding radiologist followed my stretcher out and said he was sorry to have been the one to find my trouble. His kindness was startling in its newness."[11]
>
> Tessa Carr: "A moment of exquisite human kindness: My surgeon stands beside my gurney suited in his green scrub armor, wearing his shell necklace, and gently strokes my arm as I fade away."[12]
>
> Jill Taylor: "I remember that a kind-hearted paramedic accompanied me along my journey. With compassion, he wrapped me in a blanket and arranged a jacket over my face to protect my eyes. His touch upon my back was comforting; his gentle kindness, priceless."[13]

Here in the very briefest of interactions, in each case between two strangers, recognition is established, kindness offered. We go now to slightly longer interactions, but still quite short by most any standard.

> I phoned Mr. R. W. of Harley Street, who said he would see me the next day. I presented myself hopefully, but with no particular expectations. He was a ruddy, genial man, who immediately put me at my ease, and listened with attention, occasionally asking a penetrating question. He gave me the sense that he was interested in *me*—me as a person, no less than as a problem; and he seemed to have all the time in the world, though I knew he was one of the most sought-after men in England.[14]

Busy but able to establish quickly a sense of ample time. Someone who "listened with attention" and quickly developed a specific interest in his patient.

This kind of attention is also possible in the teaching hospital. Jill Taylor recounts the first visit of a renowned neurologist doing rounds with her students:

> When she approached, she immediately reached for my foot—much like a good horse handler will touch a horse on their backside as they pass behind it. Dr. Young helped me into a comfortable position.

First, a series of gentle and strategic touches to align the bodies of the practitioner and the patient. And next, postures offering protection and making possible quite focused attention on the patient.

> She then stood by my shoulder, gently resting her hands on my arm, and spoke softly to me—not to her students, but to me. She leaned over the edge of my bed and got close enough to my face that I could hear her. Although I could not completely understand her words, I completely understood her intention.

And then a few small movements to bring closure.

> Dr. Young did not leave my bedside until she was confident that I had no more need of her. On her way out the door, she squeezed my hand and then my toe. I felt a huge sense of relief that she was my physician. I felt that she understood me.[15]

At the end, the patient feels seen and understood, though almost no technical information, indeed no words, had passed between them due to the impact of Taylor's stroke. And all this happened with small behaviors folded into customary and habitual examination movements that would lengthen (or "delay") the attending's visit no more than a minute or two.

In more serious encounters that occur within one-time or short-term relationships, it remains the case that patient narratives single out for comment precisely this matter of truly recognizing the illness at hand.

Even though my worst fears were realized in what he said [that Frank might have cancer], the physician showed, just by the way he looked at me and a couple of phrases he used, that he shared in the seriousness of my situation. The vitality of his support was as personal as it was professional.[16]

Again, notice that no huge amount of time is involved. And this from a sports medicine doctor Frank saw one time, presenting with a symptom of "back pain."

And it turns out that Broyard's desired metaphysical moment can be reached in a single comment by a practitioner with open eyes and ready compassion:

I miss [my breast], but there is something growing in its place. And it is not a tougher skin. The doctor says my heart is more exposed now. Closer to the air. "You don't have any protective tissue," she says. "I hardly need a stethoscope to hear it beat."[17]

Not only does this practitioner address the illness, and the experience of a dramatically altered body, she offers a transforming interpretation of the illness: "The surgery, the loss of your breast, has brought your heart closer to the world. This is your new life, one with your heart virtually out into the world."

The multilayered complexity, crossing through layers of time and memory, delving into the mysteries of fathers and sons of even the simplest act of the practitioner is beautifully and fearfully expressed in this poem by Mark Smith-Soto. This scene of astonishing intimacy takes place just after his surgery for prostate cancer.

Intensive Care
Your surgeon touches you like a father changing
His son, swabs, scoops, wipes around your groin,
Is this tender? Is this swollen? Is this inflamed?
His fingers run the track of his incision
To see it's zippered all the way, then satisfied

He pulls your bedclothes up, leans back
And smiles at you. Only then you realize
How carefully you've been keeping track,
Like a boy who lets his father touch him,
A father who has that right but never uses it
Except this once, this emergency when
It's a thing a man understands the secrets of,
A father thing. It may not cure you but
It heals what it heals. And you call it love.[18]

Such simple acts initiating and accomplishing healing on so many levels. Never is the body, any part of the body, "just one thing." Thus it is not correct to say that touching the body can lead the practitioner into the patient's world. Everywhere and always, the body is the lived root of the world, of every layer and facet of one's world. Touching any place on the body is touching all that is, or has been, or will be rooted in that spot. Including the complexities of body between fathers and sons.

And, finally, there's Frank's surgeon recommending a very risky biopsy procedure. After reviewing all the information and explaining the options, the surgeon says, simply, "I'm very concerned."

The way he looked at us and said "I'm very concerned" left no doubt that he was speaking as a person, not just as a medical investigator describing a case.... In that moment he became the person I wanted to have operate on me.... Being able to make those few seconds count as they did had taken him a whole life of preparing to be a person who was genuinely concerned and could express that.[19]

What a powerful notion: A lifetime of formation to become someone who could and would be that present for just a few seconds. It is at once startling and humbling.

And what about deciding which practitioner could be approached initially? One patient, asked to describe the process she used to choose practitioners she'd continued "to be loyal to" over a period of years, offered two examples:

1) Her ophthalmologist—Patient: "He answered his phone." Interviewer (puzzled): "And *that* did it?" Patient: "He said his staff was busy helping patients, and the phone was ringing, so he picked it up. The only question I had for him then was when the next open appointment was."

Aware of his context and not stuck on himself or his role. And thus likely, she assumed, to be a clinician open to recognizing and interacting with his patients.

2) Her diabetes nurse practitioner—Patient: "She opened the cabinet over her desk, sorted through several options, pulled out a new meter and handed it to me saying: 'It's the new B. B. King model.'" Interviewer (puzzled once more): "B. B. King?" Patient: "Right. My old meter was lots of trouble to use, and besides it looked like something an old guy on a surfboard might use."

In tune with her patient's culture, age, and likely preferences. Trusting the patient's assessment of the technology. No judgments, no evasions. And a dose of playful imagination! And in neither case was it technical competence that was decisive. What initiated the relationship was that one human being was recognized as a person with a full life by another.

The opposite end of "choosing one's practitioner" is the emergency room. One gets who one is given, with the resulting encounters typically anywhere from brusque to traumatic. But here is Broyard:

I found an interesting exception to this distance between the doctor and the patient. It was in the emergency room of a hospital, of all places.[20]

Broyard then describes coming into the ER in the middle of the night to get his catheter flushed and how he was received "with warm sympathy by a young intern and a beautiful nurse." And then there was the supervising physician who had recognized Broyard's name from the newspaper he worked for. His care was excellent, and they listened to his "dithyrambic account of what it felt like to empty my bladder." And then he muses:

> I think it was because it was the *emergency* room, in the front lines of medicine. These doctors and nurses still saw illness as an emergency, an emotional crisis. Also, they would meet me only once: I was a novelty, there was no question of their being permanently saddled with me. Every case in the emergency room is, in this sense, unique.... I was not so much a patient as a needy person coming in from the street. For all its occasional horrors, the emergency room is like a medical game, a continual improvisation.[21]

Yet, as many can attest, it is possible to be ignored for hours at a time in an emergency room, or treated as brusquely and speedily as possible as the backlog increases. But what is interesting here is Broyard's suggestion that a medicine that is close to the street, not buffered in offices or hospitals or research centers, might be able to see itself within the rhythms of the concrete world of patients' lives and the eruptions in those lives.

THE TRAUMA OF CARE

Much has been made in many forums of negative patient experiences in the American healthcare system and within the domains of biomedicine. We want to touch briefly here on a few negative encounters our patient authors had, because they serve as particularly graphic depictions of why recognition of and engagement with the patient as an inhabitant of a larger world are so important.

Simple callousness is an all-too-common occurrence. But then there is the phenomenon of not just being ignored, but being assaulted. These encounters constitute a significant part of what has been called "the trauma of care"—distinct from, though parallel to, the trauma of the illness. The assault is often brief, unexpected, and essentially inexplicable.

Linda Park-Fuller, writing in a performance piece, gives a first glimpse of brutality:

> SURGEON: "The other option is a lumpectomy where we remove the tumor but leave the breast. But, well, it's really not an option in your case, because the tumor is so large and your breasts are so small."
> SHE: (To audience): "Huh! 'Insult to injury' wouldn't you say?" (Stands, crosses stage.)

This is a technical description but also a personal insult. And the insult directed to just that very part of Park-Fuller's body-self, her breast, that was already suffering and vulnerable. And, by virtue of being a woman's breast in our contemporary culture, already over-charged, objectified, subject to scrutiny.[22]

Kay Jamison, author of one of the standard textbooks on manic-depressive illness, goes in to consult a psychiatrist for treatment of her own manic-depression. He does a thorough history and then asks if she plans to have children. And in doing so asks if she knows that manic-depression is a genetic disease. She responds that, yes, she knows this (!), and goes on to make comments about lithium and pregnancy, and to say that she very much wants to have children.

> At that point, in an icy and imperious voice that I can hear to this day, he stated—as though it were God's truth, which he no doubt felt that it was—"You shouldn't have children. You have manic-depressive illness." I felt sick, unbelievably and utterly sick, and deeply humiliated.

Later, reflecting on the fact that she had never regretted having been born, she realizes it had never occurred to her not to have children because of her illness.

Brutality takes many forms, and what he had done was not only brutal but unprofessional and uninformed. It did the kind of lasting damage that only something that cuts so quick and deep to the heart can do.

These are blows to the body-self, to the self-image, and they have a personal edge.[23]

Race, blackness, combined with gender, opens the patient to very distinctive forms of personal negation. And this can be the case even when the patient is herself a physician:

> I had twin babies; I was on maternity leave. I took them to a urologist that my pediatrician recommended. And, you know, I had my hair pulled back in a ponytail, and I had on a university sweatshirt with blue jeans, and when the guy walked in, the first thing he asked me was, "Are you married?" He didn't introduce himself. He didn't say, "Hi. I'm Dr. So-and-so. I hear you . . . " The very first thing out of his mouth was, "Are you married?"

There is the basic rudeness, first of all. No introduction, no connection. A physician who bluntly jumps right in to make an assessment based on racism: "Young black women with twins." And an assessment that in any case has nothing to do with the matter at hand. And so it becomes an impromptu, uninvited, and unwanted editorial on culture, race, and economics. Blindness; an attack on all African Americans, and doubly so on African-American women; and a direct personal insult. All "accomplished" in the time it took to walk into the room and ask one question.

> So I just explained in medical terms why I was here to see him. I didn't even answer his question. I just used medical terms for everything. And he goes, "Who are you?" I said, "I'm an attending physician at _____." And he goes, "Oh. I went to _____." I have no idea why that came out of his mouth, it was just really disappointing. But it did illustrate to me, the fact that I continued

to let him do the surgery on my son, how powerful physicians are. Plenty of people could have done that surgery, and I let him do it. I still don't understand why I did that. And how weak I was. I didn't feel like a doctor at the time—I felt like an overworked mother of twins, you know?

Negotiations of interpersonal power happen frighteningly quickly. Decades and decades of the conditioning of individuals and of social groups are brought to bear on such situations instantaneously. And all of that lies behind physicians as they complete even the simplest interactions with patients.

Other times the blows are not so very personal and so very social, but serve rather to enforce an anonymity or objectification that has a brutality all its own. Reynolds Price is lying on a gurney in the hallway. Two doctors approach him with results from a battery of tests.

> But all I recall the two men saying that instant, then and there in the hallway mob scene, was "The upper ten or twelve inches of your spinal cord have swelled and are crowding the available space. The cause could be a tumor . . . "

They say they'll have a promising young neurosurgeon come by and then walk off, leaving Price and his brother still in the hall "stared at by strangers."[24] This is the logical concomitant of "the tumor on gurney number 5." The physiologically abstracted body is given abstracted physiological information. Tumor, spinal cord, pressure, surgery. Next.

In many less egregious cases, it is the quick alternation of the positive and the negative that highlights each. This is Jill Taylor speaking about her second day in the hospital after her stroke:

> I awoke early the next morning to a medical student who came rushing in to take a medical history. . . . This young girl was an energy vampire. She wanted to take something from me despite my fragile condition, and she had nothing to give me in return.

She was rushing against a clock and obviously losing the race. In her haste, she was rough in the way she handled me. . . . She spoke a million miles a minute and hollered at me as if I were deaf.[25]

And then later the same day another medical student comes by to do one more neurological exam:

I was wobbly, incredibly weak, and not capable of sitting up by myself. . . . But because he was gentle yet firm in his touch, I felt safe with him. He spoke calmly, looked me directly in the eyes, and repeated himself as needed. He was respectful of me as a person—even in this condition.[26]

The enormous difference a change in stance and intent can make. And changing from one to the other could be so simple: slowing down, being gentle and calm, looking directly into the eyes. The small things provide safety and offer the recognition of one human being by another.

And then there are forms of negation that unfold more slowly. For a patient, being misdiagnosed is not simply, or primarily, a technical failure—a failure of skill or failure to apply a skill effectively; it is a failure of recognition. Take Susan Miller's experience—which is not, unfortunately, atypical. Her partner finds a lump in her breast, a lump that turns out to be a malignant tumor. Her gynecologist tells her it's a gland. But the lump doesn't go away, so that doctor sends her to a surgeon in Los Angeles, who tells her it's a fibroadenoma. "Someday you might want to have it removed. But no rush. It's benign." The lump continues to grow. In New York she consults another surgeon, who asks what she has been told so far. After she goes through her history, he says: "I'm concerned. I want to biopsy it right now."[27]

Penetrating diagnosis is thought of so often as a stellar example of a purely technical skill, and there is no doubt that technical skill and scientific knowledge are essential ingredients in making an accurate diagnosis. But much of diagnosis involves paying attention to the patient as she lives in her world. Thus, being misdiagnosed is an experience of not being seen, of not being heard or listened to or taken seriously. It is also at times a negation, a condescending judgment on the patient's basic competence as a human being, or on her adequacy as a moral agent. All great diagnosticians know this.

Tessa Carr gives a particularly thorough account of the impact continual invisibility has on her life as she goes to doctor after doctor on the way to being diagnosed, finally, with a tumor of her adrenal glands.[28] The important point is not that she was misdiagnosed regularly over a period of two full years, a typically fatal condition being overlooked again and again. These basic facts do certainly convey a dramatic and terrifying life-rupturing. But it is the ongoing assault on and negation of the patient accompanying the misdiagnoses that warrant our special attention here. Let us begin with something many patients complain about, the delivery of bad news: "While I am standing in an airport, I receive a call that tells me that the inside of my body from chest to pelvis must be scanned to find the tumor or tumors." And another call about test results: "I find out that I have fatal levels of adrenaline circulating in my body every day."[29]

It is as though speaking such news face to face, and sitting with the shock and initial grief, is simply too much. (Recall Price's experience in the hallway, described earlier.) And so the messenger becomes a staff person, not the physician. And all too often, it is the phone that is the medium through which the bad news is delivered.

And then there is the matter of having been seen by a battery of physicians. In Carr's case this included a university health center doctor; an internist; an ER doctor; a neurologist; a chiropractor; and another neurologist. It was the second neurologist who made the full diagnosis. And finally a surgical oncologist and endocrinologist treats the disease without engaging the illness. Her presenting symptoms are intermittent and include pallor, irregular heart rate, high blood pressure, and a sense of impending doom. During her trip through these various physician offices these symptoms are progressing to: unbreakable migraines, projectile vomiting, shaking, and muscle contractions. And throughout this she has, of course, undergone test after test of major bodily systems: CT scans, MRIs, ultrasounds, and blood tests. And then, at long last, the second neurologist schedules tests of her adrenal levels.

But meanwhile, and most insultingly, there is the running commentary of her practitioners on her competence as a human being—on what, to use an old-fashioned word, can only be called her character.

- University health center physician, on Carr's first visit: "You need to relax, you need to get this blood pressure under control. We're starting you on some medication but you should be exercising to bring your blood pressure down. I know your comps are stressful, but you have to manage that pressure."
- University health center physician, responding to a phone call about a blood pressure reading of 220/140: "Your cuff must be wrong."

Translation: "You're not managing your life well. And you're a bit hysterical. Your evaluation of your condition means nothing, as you're likely a somatizer."

- Neurologist: [He] pronounces that the year's worth of testing I had undergone with other doctors was worthless. I only have "classic migraine" disorder. He discontinues my blood pressure medications. "Migraine is a condition that you manage for life."

Translation: "Because you, in your weakness, have not managed your migraine, you have led your doctors to order an entire year of worthless tests. But I have found you out. You must buck up—life is hard. Deal with your pain. Manage your migraine."[30]

And what does the world of her illness look like as she continues through this set of encounters? Carr's ability to work and maintain a regular schedule are lost. And then there was the internal part of the illness:

The feeling was one of disintegration, a fine and quick breaking apart. . . . The pain that resonated through my body was not as unbearable as the constant fear for my sanity. [This] brings the saddest memories of loneliness.[31]

Finally, the second neurologist consults with the original internist, and the tests of the adrenal glands are ordered. This leads to the phone call in the airport. And next:

> I am immediately referred to a surgical oncologist and subsequently an endocrinologist. I have what is most likely a "benign" adrenaline-producing tumor called a "pheochromocytoma." It is enraging to finally feel vindicated because someone has told me what I knew all along—I am very close to death.[32]

The surgical oncologist later confides to her that endocrinologists wait their entire careers to see a case like hers.

What from the clinician's point of view may be taken up as a series of technical errors is inevitably, most emphatically experienced by patients as something very personal, as a compounding of the risk to and the illness of their complete life-world. "My world cannot be restored, because I wasn't seen." And not being seen is not just about some "emotional need" of a particular patient or the "psychological dynamic" in a particular case that the practitioner must somehow "handle." It is, often enough, a matter of living and dying.

Arthur Frank found a ridge on his left testicle. He goes to his doctor and is told it's chlamydia, a disease he says was unknown to him. He's offered penicillin—but no questions about sexual partners, no warnings about future sexual activities, and no information about the far more dire consequences for women of such an infection. The penicillin didn't help, so he was given another course of it. Then came back pain, so he returned to his doctor, who switched his medicine to sulfa, saying penicillin sometimes caused back pain. He has a reaction to the sulfa, so the doctor takes him off all medications and refers him to a urologist, who can see him in two months. The back pain gets so bad he goes to the ER, where he is diagnosed as "chronically constipated." Still troubled by the back pain, he goes to see a sports medicine specialist. And it is this man who makes the initial diagnosis. This was fortunate, given that testicular cancer is one of the fastest-growing cancers, and cure rates vary directly with early detection.[33]

Once more we are being told of one of the most frustrating and at times terrifying experiences in contemporary biomedicine: having one specialist after another say, "No, in my portion of the body-sphere, I can't name what you have. Whatever it is, it's not in my word-box. Try the guy in the next booth." Or, "Yes, this fits in my space. It's called chlamydia, and here's your penicillin for it." Or, again, "Yes, this fits in my space and here it is—a prescription for your constipation." (Which both Carr and Frank received.) As though the hope is that the patient will move on to another place with the problem.

The additional point here is that rather than bringing the latest of scientific research to bear on a particular system of the body, specialization threatens to become, in contemporary practice, a refusal of the responsibility to name. Or a narrowing down that is so dramatic that it becomes a refusal. Rapid-fire triage.

HEALING OVER THE LONG TERM

The achievement of trust and confidence in short-term interactions between patients and practitioners can open into long-term relationships that are healing and in the long run mutually beneficial. These longer-term relationships engage those deeper resources of patient and practitioner that can only be accessed over time, as a shared body of experience is built between them. They allow the development of a moral complexity and subtlety that the short-term interactions preclude. The person who becomes a patient's long-term practitioner comes to see and to share in more and more facets of the patient's world. And the practitioners most appreciated are the ones who tailor care and treatment to their patient's capabilities and priorities, in whatever way that is possible.

For short-term care, DO THIS:

- Greet me as people typically greet each other: look at me, slow down, be polite, listen to me.
- Speak to me, and not about me to others in the room.
- Recognize that I am in a life crisis when I come to you. Make room for this experience in our interaction—a matter of *perception*: "I see." Empathy. Acknowledge seriousness when that's appropriate.
- Invite me to be a partner in my own healing. Take seriously my account of my illness. Tell me the truth.
- Acknowledge that I have a world and a life outside the exam room, outside the hospital.
- Be calm. Make some kind of gentle physical contact to reassure my wounded body.
- Use humor and imagination to open up tight spaces.
- Be careful how you name or label my condition. That name or label will carry much weight with me and my caregivers, and it will follow me all the way through the medical system.
- Keep me in your sight. I want to be visible.

For short-term care, DON'T DO THIS:

- Be in a hurry or distracted.
- Speak rapidly, in jargon, without pausing.
- Focus only on my disease.
- Deliver enormously consequential information brusquely, quickly, and/or in public locations.
- Discredit my statements about my condition.
- Be rude or callous in dealing with me and my primary caregivers.
- Insult my capabilities or my intelligence—or my race, gender, social class, or religion.
- Drain my energy. Subject me to exhausting procedures, especially if they are of less than critical importance, and especially when I am still weak from initial trauma.
- Spend more time at your computer or consulting your formulary than you do looking at me and talking to me.
- Make me invisible. Drop me or ignore me or look away.

The long-term relationship between patient and provider typically begins with a strong sense of affirmation of the patient's illness, and of the crisis in the patient's world, by the provider:

I had seen seven doctors and had had dozens of tests, including a heart cath, over a two-month period before I decided to try an acupuncturist. What I recall most clearly now is that my acupuncturist had a name for something that the physicians did not. I honestly didn't understand the name—something about being warm when I should be cold—or cool when I should be warm. And something about my hollow organs and my solid ones, and then disturbances in my pulses (plural). But I trusted her naming because she listened to me for 45 minutes in that first appointment.

A process is begun of actually looking at what was going on in this patient's world and body, and seeing what was found as unique.

She sat on a stool that put her at just my eye level, and looked me in the eye that whole time. I was fully clothed during all this—no gown, no "take your shirt off before the doctor comes in." She took copious notes. She was confident. I thought to myself that I had finally found someone who would stand by me in this, whatever it is. True, after that she stuck me with needles and sent me home to brew the most awful-smelling, awful-tasting concoction I've ever consumed. Whatever it was, I began to eat again. I gained back some of the 20–30 pounds I'd lost. And, most important, I finally had some hope.

The long-term practitioners tend to be the "diagnosing" clinician, and are quite often not the first practitioner seen. The "breakthrough" practitioner is the one who does not simply apply familiar and convenient labels common in her specialty or modality. This practitioner is the one who recognizes fully the nature of the crisis occurring in the patient's world. And this is, from the patient's point of view, as much if not more a matter of actually listening to and believing and trusting the patient, as it is a matter of technical skill or expertise.

Practitioners involved in the long-term relationship consistently acknowledge that the patient's primary life and world lie outside the domain of the medical system within which they practice—whether that medical system be allopathic, Ayurvedic, Chinese, or homeopathic. And, further, they recognize that the resources contained in that "nonmedicalized" world are essential aspects of the patient's healing process, equally as important for the healing of illness as clinical interventions.[34]

An admittedly unusual but nonetheless instructive example here is the practitioner who treated Norman Cousins's illness, based on their existing 20-year relationship. This physician helps him move from the hospital to a motel so Cousins can escape an environment he believes is draining his energy and working primarily to assault the healing resources he has left, the most prominent of which is sleep. The motel setting also allows Cousins continuously to watch the slapstick comedies and engage in the deep laughter that help relieve his pain and keep his emotions positive—and that help him, in Cousins's own account, overcome the poisoning going on within his body. This same physician, though somewhat skeptical or even alarmed, goes along with Cousins's ideas about extraordinarily intense vitamin C therapy, intended once more to combat the disintegration of connective tissue that is at the core of Cousins's illness.

> I was incredibly fortunate to have as my doctor a man who knew that his biggest job was to encourage to the fullest the patient's will to live and to mobilize all the natural resources of body and mind to combat disease.[35]

It is important to note that Cousins and his physician had been "close friends for over 20 years," so a sound, solid foundation of mutual trust and respect had already been constructed. Drawing on this existing long-term relationship, they were able to effect an extraordinary recovery from what was diagnosed at that time as ankylosing spondylitis. And one can only imagine the increased power and clarity that joint experience brought into an already remarkable relationship. Engaging the patient's full resources is, as we will discuss below, one of the traits most appreciated by patients in long-term relationship with their practitioners.[36]

Long-term healing relationships are based on the determination and the ability of both clinician and the patient to stay the course, no matter what twists and turns occur as the illness progresses. Laced through and animating this commitment not to abandon the patient is the shared confidence that the patient can get better, can live a fuller life. And that the effort necessary to make that happen—on the part of the practitioner and the patient—is absolutely worthwhile. Kay Jamison speaks eloquently of this in her description of her psychiatrist:

> The debt I owe my psychiatrist is beyond description. I remember sitting in his office a hundred times during those grim months and each time thinking, What on earth can he say that will make me feel better or keep me alive? Well, there never was anything he could say, that's the funny thing. It was all the stupid, desperately optimistic, condescending things he *didn't* say that kept me alive; all the compassion and warmth I felt from him that could not have been said; all the intelligence, competence, and time he put into it; and *his granite belief that mine was a life worth living.*[37]

It is not just that extraordinary practitioners keep their own confidence in the healing process. They continue to reach out into their patients' despair and fear and lack of confidence to reengage them in the healing partnership.

> He was terribly direct, which was terribly important, and he was willing to admit the limits of his understanding and treatments and when he was wrong.[38]

And then there is truth-telling, a foundational element in long-term relationships and arrangements of all kinds. But the quality of truth-telling involved in practitioner–patient relationships goes to a different level, driven there by the severity of the crisis in the patient's body-world. Such radical truth-telling is the critical precondition for the confidence-building of which we were just speaking.

Reynolds Price has similar things to say about the surgeon who saves his life. The surgeon stays with him through operation after operation, through each experiment with each innovative technology. And all this in spite of his own doubts that Price will make it through. The relationship begins simply and quietly, but solidly: "Friedman stopped by twice a day; and unlike most members of the senior staff in a teaching hospital, he never arrived with a guard of students. He came alone with his own intense focus . . . "[39] As the bond between them grows, Price speaks of Friedman describing the cells in the tumor with "a kind of aesthetic frown." And then, two years later, there is Friedman's real delight when, using a new laser surgery technique in two different operations, he makes enormous advances in removing quantities of tumor from Price's spine.

> Friedman claims with great satisfaction—"We're way ahead of the game." . . . I noted his first-time use of the *we* and began comprehending the stake he'd had in my case from the very start when he'd foreseen a thoroughly dark outcome.

The mutuality, the shared stake in overcoming the ongoing crisis of Price's life, is now so very evident. And this allows Price to take the next step and go beyond recognizing Friedman's qualities as a practitioner and a surgeon, and to grasp him more fully as a human being.

> By now I could see that his satisfaction was far more nearly that of a well-meant fellow creature than a self-respecting virtuoso; and I wished I'd had the self-possession two years before to see his shy phone calls for what they were—offers of friendship, not grist for his files.[40]

Here we have come full circle, from the practitioner recognizing the patient as a person inhabiting a life-world in crisis that is far larger than the person found in the medical system, to the patient recognizing the physician as a person inhabiting a life-world far larger than the clinician found within the medical system.[41] And, finally, this is what both patients and practitioners long for. It is the deep wellspring of their mutual healing.

As we might expect from first-person accounts, from memoirs such as these, there is great emphasis on the patient's own role in her healing. While some of this may be attributed to presentation of self and our natural egotism, the core turns out to be a common theme. The patient, and particularly the patient given a very dire diagnosis and prognosis, comes to realize: "I am the one who has to make the recovery happen. I am the one who has final, fundamental, and primary responsibility for my own healing." Jill Taylor, Reynolds Price, and Norman Cousins all describe making this decisive interior movement. And then the further realization: "Clinicians can help me, and that help is essential. But finally it is my job." In each case, the patient making this movement reports a dramatic turn for the better as this realization comes to permeate their entire being. And this was so even if it meant looking squarely at his or her own death, as it did for Broyard.

Practitioners who develop relationships that heal over the long term recognize that they play the decisive role in endorsing, affirming, and validating the patient's central role in their own healing. Or to put it in the imperative, "Amplify your own good work by affirming the patient's power to act and to heal." In addition, patients encouraged to step up and take charge will typically stop expecting their clinician to do all the healing work. Or more bluntly, in terms that may seem self-serving, even minimal engagement of the patient in his or her own healing reduces the practitioner's burden. Building relationships with patients is the key to preventing burnout, not the primary cause of it.

Harold Brodkey's relationship with his practitioner provides an outstanding example of all the elements composing long-term healing relationships that we've been reviewing. Brodkey is diagnosed with AIDS in spring 1993, and this is when he meets his new doctor, Barry Hartman, an infectious disease specialist.[42] Hartman will stay with Brodkey through the course of his disease, until he dies in fall 1995. Hartman explains aspects of the new world of AIDS that Brodkey is entering. And, in turn, he listens—and negotiates—as Brodkey struggles with his medications and all the other challenges facing the newly diagnosed AIDS patient. A particularly telling moment comes that first spring when Brodkey tells Hartman he "can't hack it here" in the hospital, that he has to get out, has to attend to his life—and he has to *write*. Hartman is puzzled by this, noting that Brodkey has a "peculiar attitude" towards AIDS and towards death. But he listens. And then he convinces Brodkey to stay a bit longer in the hospital to complete some more therapies for the pneumonia, taper off some medications, and do the inevitable additional round of tests. And then Hartman begins giving advice on living outside the hospital: on universal precautions and keeping gloves handy, on not buying his AIDS medicines at his local drugstore but at a "discreet" shop, because if the people in his neighborhood knew about his condition, they would treat him differently, badly. Ellen Brodkey, Harold's wife, asks Hartman questions about nutrition and proper diet. To Harold Brodkey's delight Hartman responds, "I want him to gain weight, no matter what it takes." He wants Harold not to "be surprised if you can't *do* much at first. But hang on." Hartman is worried about the medical problems, yes. And so he explains to Harold and Ellen what he can do in terms of medicines to keep him relatively healthy. "You should start on AZT now." But he also wants to assist Harold and his primary caregiver, Ellen, as they struggle to live the illness as fully as they can. As Harold put it, "Barry changed in his own notions about what was best for me; he saw it more and more in terms of us."[43]

And, in fact, Harold gradually recovers and is finally far stronger when he has been out of the hospital six months. And Hartman is large enough to acknowledge this and continues to support the couple's choices. This fidelity and openness to the patient's actual life-experience is what our patients all want to find.

And at the end, Harold displays in his writing a remarkable healing and clarity, a startling, lean wholeness:

I don't want any human gesture of solidarity. I feel quite human anyway, infinitely human, which is to say merely human, and I don't feel the need for physical reassurance. I find the silence of God to be very beautiful, even when the silence is directed at me.[44]

Cantankerous to the end, but resolved and reconciled:

Peace? There was never any in the world. But in the pliable water, under the sky, unmoored, I am traveling now and hearing myself laugh, at first with nerves and then with genuine amazement. It is all around me.[45]

And how much of this can we attribute to the quality of care and attention and compassion his doctor and his wife offered Harold in his last year? An unanswerable question. But if one compares the Harold who is writing at the beginning of this memoir to the Harold who is writing at the end, one would be inclined to argue that their contribution must have been considerable.

Ellen's central and utterly essential role in Harold's illness—and what can only be called his healing by dying—demonstrates eloquently how crucial the care is that is offered by the person who becomes the primary caregiver when the patient's life-world breaks apart. Which, of course, for spouse or partner or family member, means a rupturing of their own world as well. The primary caregiver then is expected to deal with his own often considerable loss while also being the primary healing resource for the patient. It is no wonder that the central role of this person in the patient's healing, and the healing of the crisis in patient's body-world, is a key theme in account after account. The primary caregivers take on a wide range of duties and responsibilities. They help recall technical information received from healthcare providers that the patient cannot recall or often understand, because of medications or trauma or the sheer amount of information delivered in a short piece of time. And then there are the conversations afterward with the patient trying to sort through this complex information, figure out which new questions to ask, and make any decisions necessary at this point. And these discussions are seldom simple and often contentious, as the patient struggles to maintain some rudiments of autonomy and dignity, and is yet relying completely on, and being mostly grateful for, the assistance the caregiver is providing. And then there is what may be considered the complementary function of being the expert on who the patient is, what their life is about, what is important to them, their medical history, and the circumstances surrounding the onset of the illness.

The primary caregiver is also expected to manage the inevitable, but often unexpected, new blows or traumas that health care and the turns of an illness always seem to entail. And to provide emotional support during such reverses, and afterward. And finally there is the day-to-day "stuff": cleaning the bathroom being used by someone who often has little control over his urination or defecation. Keeping clothes clean, disinfecting items that come home from the hospital, changing dressings, giving baths, buying and cooking food while considering special dietary needs of the patient, and on to helping the patient negotiate with employers or clients. It is a matter, finally, of living two lives at once. And one of the critical responsibilities of the practitioner is to empower and support such caregivers. To protect them as a valuable resource—and sometimes protect them, if the clinician is paying careful enough attention, from their patient. The cost here can be enormous. As Arthur Frank says candidly,

> But the intensity of illness also burned out something in that relationship [his marriage]. Those three years were a time when each of us needed so much, and most of it had to come from the other partner, who was equally needy. *We have never fully recovered.*[46]

And yet, as our accounts document, time after time people step into this critical role, into this place of responsibility and sacrifice.

For Brodkey and Frank it is their spouses. For Carr it is her spouse and her sister. For Price it is his brother and a community of friends. For Taylor it is her mother, who climbs into the bed with Taylor when first arriving at the hospital and spends years with Taylor as caregiver, stand-in physical therapist and speech therapist, and loving companion.[47]

And there is Nancy Mairs's daughter. Mairs is cooking dinner and her daughter is reading close by:

> As I opened a can of tomatoes, the can slipped in my left hand and juice splattered me and the counter with bloody spots. Fatigued and infuriated, I bellowed, "I'm so sick of being crippled!" [Mairs has MS.] Anne glanced at me over the top of her book. "There now," she said, "do you feel better?" "Yes," I said, "yes, I do." She went back to her reading. I felt better. That's about all the attention my scurviness ever gets.[48]

For Audre Lorde it is a small, tightly bound community of women:

> I do know that there was a tremendous amount of love and support flowing into me from the women around me, and it felt like being bathed in a continuous tide of positive energies.[49]

The degree of connectedness in this group was strong enough to reach into Lorde's own identity:

> To this day, *sometimes I feel like a corporate effort*, the love and care and concern of so many women having been invested in me with such open-heartedness.[50]

This sense of identity shaped by, flowing out of others—a marriage, a family, a community—is such a resource for healing of unimaginable richness. Lorde's summarizing formulation puts it perfectly: "Perhaps I can say this all more simply; the love of women healed me."[51]

For the practitioner, fully engaging the patient's world must include engaging the patient's primary caregivers. It is important for the clinician to know what resources they have to offer and to see the limits of what they can offer. And sometimes it is necessary for the practitioner to help the patient see these limits, which the patient often cannot—because of the nature of the crisis and its treatment, because of pain or medications or a basic bewilderment. The primary caregivers are potentially one of the clinician's most potent healing resources and should be cultivated accordingly.

For long-term care, DO THIS:

- See me first—not your diagnostic system, or the diagnostic label(s) you receive from other practitioners.
- Fidelity. Be faithful. Stay with me and consistently reassure me about this.
- Tell me the truth.
- My engagement over the long haul is key: Keep me going. Work with me to overcome discouragement, fear, despair—and any blocks that arise in our relationship.
- Affirm my grasp of and stance towards my illness. This is the foundation of all else.
- My primary caregivers are essential. Keep them engaged over the long haul.
- In the course of long-term care, your staff and support people (PAs, RNs, therapists, social workers, aides, insurance clerks, and receptionists) will spend more time with me than you will. Make sure they're attentive, kind, and well trained.
- Be open to knowing me and my world more fully.
- Be open to having me know you more fully, as a practitioner and as a human being.

For long-term care, DON'T DO THIS:

- Refuse to recognize me as human as things go on and on and on.
- Protect me from the truth, by omission or evasion or fabrication.
- Let my care become routinized.
- Stop seeing me—especially if I am getting worse and approaching being "incurable."
- Abandon me.

RENEWAL

There are those fortunate times when a long-term relationship calls for the practitioner to participate in the patient's efforts to build a new world for himself, to construct a new life. This can be immensely gratifying and nourishing for the practitioner, and completely renewing for the patient. And this renewal may well take place where the hoped-for healing has not taken place, when the practitioner may feel he has failed or achieved only "limited success." But the healing that can happen at just this point is the drawing of a larger circle, a shift in perspective, the discovery of new goals. And clinicians must trust that this is possible. Both the practitioner and the patient must trust that *a person's life has its own trajectory that is far more powerful than any medicine*.

And it is, in fact, a common theme in our accounts that patients often experience their lives as far richer and fuller after their severe illnesses, and on account of those illnesses. Even illness that results in dramatic changes in the old world: Price as paraplegic; Mairs with MS.

> This gentleness is part of the reason that I'm not sorry to be a cripple. I didn't have it before.... It has opened and enriched my life enormously, this sense that my frailty and need must be mirrored in others, that in searching for and shaping a stable core in a life wrenched by change and loss, change and loss, I must recognize the same process, under individual conditions, in the lives around me.[52]

Brodkey moving toward his death, as we saw above. And Broyard toward his:

> My body, which in the last decade or two had become a familiar, no-longer-thrilling old flame, was reborn as a brand-new infatuation. I realize of course that this elation I feel is just a phase, just a rush of consciousness, a splash of perspective, a hot flash of ontological alertness. But I'll take it, I'll use it.[53]

A facet of one's self pulled forward—"gentleness." The body's magic rediscovered. The textures and contours of living illuminated:

> The ultimate value of illness is that it teaches us the value of being alive; this is why the ill are not just charity cases, but a presence to be valued. . . . Illness restores the sense of proportion that is lost when we take life for granted.[54]

Lorde gives it to us very succinctly: "I would never have chosen this path, but I am very glad to be who I am, here."[55] It is the fortunate practitioner, the one who has been loyal and committed and deeply giving, who is presented with the opportunity to participate in this ultimate level of healing that illness can offer.

NOT SAINTHOOD, BUT SIMPLE HUMANITY

When you actually look at what makes a difference for patients with their healthcare providers—in the beginning, especially—what you find are actions that are relatively simple and direct. Patients aren't expecting Mother Teresa, or Dr. Chekhov, or Sigmund Freud. (In fact, most of us would prefer, when we are patients, something not nearly as powerful or intrusive!) What we want is to be met as a human being by another human being who is also our healthcare practitioner.

Much of this is not complex; much of it is already there. The patient is simply asking, "Even though it may be scary, meet me as one human being to another." True, some practitioners may have fewer skills than others in building or maintaining relationships. That's clearly true in every group of people: academics, warehouse workers, truck drivers, senators. But two things may be said about that: 1) When the relatively unskilled make a true effort, that effort itself will most likely be enough to begin establishing a connection. 2) In any case, this is for sure: unless the relatively unskilled make such efforts, they'll never develop the skills that our patient accounts point to as essential.

Let us look once more at why this basic level, why the very small things are so important. Partly it is what Price speaks to so emphatically and clearly in the passage we quoted earlier in this chapter. The small things are basic aspects of any human interaction. But there is another factor that is quite specific to people who are very sick. People who are compromised, people in the midst of a world crisis, need simple things. Such things are, in many cases, all they can respond to. Normal processing is disrupted and needs to be re-established. And safety is decisive for this. As a formulation: Simplicity + Gentleness = Safety. Consequently, the more compromised the patient, the more important the simple things become in the whole scheme. Without the simple things, many patients will not go on to more complex interactions.

> It was my decision to show up or not. I chose to show up for those professionals who brought me energy by connecting with me, touching me gently and appropriately, making direct eye contact with me, and speaking to me calmly.[56]

Seldom are all functions compromised. But the path to the functions that are not compromised, or the least compromised, is through the "little things."

> The more extreme the situation, the more time and help I need to say anything. When I face someone who does not seem willing or able to help me work toward what I might eventually say, I become mute.[57]

Again, it is kindness and simplicity that make it safe enough for patients to risk bringing forward the uninjured pieces. Which are only uninjured, from patient's point of view, because they have been so well protected so far. Or, to put it differently, the intact systems are operating in an "all alert, fight-or-flight mode." And the key to getting past this is providing safety. And what provides safety is the little things.

For a practitioner to open herself emotionally 30 times a day is not possible; no one should expect that. But smiling and touching and being present should be possible a high percentage of the time. Maybe even, on a good day, 70 to 80 percent. The critical point is not numbers. The critical point is that every clinician's success in recognizing the fuller world of the patient, and in turn being recognized as a human being by the patient, is a major achievement in a biomedical system that is as brutal for clinicians as it is for patients.

As a further step towards fuller mutual recognition, one of our hospital-based clinicians suggests spending an extra 5 to 10 minutes at the end of the day with one patient seen that day. This allows the practitioner to make deeper connections while protecting himself from being overwhelmed.

Another practitioner notes that each week there will likely be some patients who draw the clinician further than usual into their world. Patients come in who somehow seem to be "sent." Situations arise where something "extra" may be asked of or elicited from the clinician, and where in turn the patient offers an unexpected blessing.

The lesson is that the minimal is so often enough yet so often beyond what is commonly given. And that this minimum provides the foundation for all the complexity that follows, both complexity in relationships and complexity of the technical skills and information the practitioner has to offer.

I may not expect emotion or intimacy from physicians and nurses, but I do expect recognition.[58]

We don't want our hospitals full of saints—everything would likely shut down. But we do want practitioners' offices and hospitals full of people who can—from time to time, maybe even most of the time—be decent human beings. For the truth of the matter is that most patients would be delighted (a) to receive a very basic level of recognition and (b) not to be traumatized by their care.

Admittedly, the biomedical healthcare system so very often makes even such basic levels of human recognition terribly difficult. But this may be turned in another direction: By being a decent human being, one becomes a hero. For, as David Hilfiker puts it, "Not all of us are saints."[59]

[6]

THE BIOLOGY OF HEALING: NEUROSCIENCE AND THE EDUCATION OF HEALERS

(with Eve Henry, M.D.)

Although many of us think of ourselves as *thinking creatures that feel*, biologically we are *feeling creatures that think*.

—Jill Bolte Taylor

In previous chapters we have given a detailed exposition of the thinking and experiences of talented clinicians, people who have exceptional relational skills and are able to establish lasting therapeutic alliances with their patients and clients. In Chapter 5 we added to this practitioner study a more limited analysis of patient perceptions of healing. In both cases the evidence we have presented is qualitative. It does not provide a biomedical model for how healing occurs. Hence, however convinced clinicians and patients may be, their practical knowledge of how compassionate and trusting interactions work may still be discounted because scientific modeling of this phenomenon lags behind practical wisdom. The aim of this chapter is to begin to address this gap.

Through the process of single and then double blinding in research, the advance of modern biomedical science has sought to exclude the confounding issue of how the mental states of both patients and physicians influence health outcomes. The advances achieved through this exclusion have been profound. Yet a growing body of research indicates that the mental states of both parties can be studied and in many cases have important and physiologically measurable healing effects. We are not, to be sure, advocating a diminished reliance on the double-blind, randomized controlled trial as a gold standard for medical science. We are simply saying that this model must be complemented by research that takes account of, rather than seeking to eliminate, the powerful impact of the quality of relationships between practitioners and their patients.

There is mounting scientific evidence that the practitioner–patient relationship is an important factor in how patients get better. Three well-known studies will help to introduce our discussion.

In an ingenious experiment Colloca, Benedetti, and colleagues devised two means for postoperative patients to receive an analgesic injection. One group was given the injection through a computer-controlled infusion pump without being told the purpose of the injection. A second group was given the analgesic by a clinician, who described the injection as a pain-relieving intervention. The differences were noteworthy. The patients given the machine-administered analgesic needed significantly higher doses to achieve the same reduction in pain, and in addition the patients who received their injections from a clinician had substantially faster pain relief.[1]

In another study Kaptchuk and colleagues followed 262 adults with irritable bowel syndrome (IBS) over a six-week period. The single-blind, randomized, controlled trial separated participants into three groups: assessment and observation, placebo acupuncture alone, or placebo acupuncture with a patient–practitioner relationship enhanced by warmth, attention, and confidence. The placebo acupuncture combined with an enhanced relationship with the practitioner provided significant improvement in IBS symptoms, while placebo acupuncture yielded only modest improvement over assessment and observation alone.[2]

These two studies are similar to the decades of research by Kiecolt-Glaser and her colleagues, who have shown that mental states can affect the immune system both positively and negatively. Their work demonstrates that stress can increase the time needed to heal a wound and that social support can aid in healing when it is present and harm the patient when it is lacking.[3]

We should not be at all surprised that mental states and cognitive activity can change physiology. It's as easily recognizable as blushing, fear-induced heart pounding, fainting at the sight of blood, and sexual arousal. We sometimes forget that these routine and well-recognized reactions are all mediated through pathways that move from thought to the neural networks of the brain and into the rest of the body. So the underlying thesis, that mental states can affect physiological processes, is uncontroversial. We have routine confirmation that thoughts and attitudes alter the body. What we are presenting below is simply a more systematic, detailed mapping of this territory, based on current research.

TOWARD A BIOMEDICAL MODEL OF HEALING RELATIONSHIPS

The context of the clinical encounter, including relational dimensions of the interaction between clinician and patient, contribute to a patient's placebo response, or what we will call "the healing response." Inherent in every clinical encounter or procedure are multiple factors that make up the psychosocial context of the event. These factors are often amorphous and difficult to describe. They can be as simple as the "feeling" a patient gets when he or she walks into the physician's office, or as complicated as a patient's entire lifetime of past medical experiences. Henry has grouped these various factors into four broad categories that have been individually shown to affect treatment outcome.[4] These categories are not the only ones that work to incite a healing response, but they are factors about which there are credible research findings. They serve as examples of how simple, often overlooked,

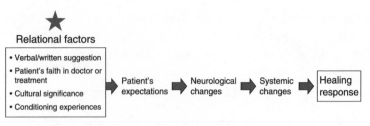

Figure 6.1

aspects of the medical encounter can create expectations within the patient that can lead to objective neurological and immunological responses that result in healing.

The four broad categories of factors within the patient–doctor interaction, as displayed in Figure 6.1, are a patient's past experiences, any verbal or written suggestions a patient encounters, the cultural significance of the treatment or diagnosis, and the patient's faith in the physician and the treatment plan.

In terms of *verbal and written suggestions*, it seems that patients heal, in part, because their physicians tell them to do so. Benedetti and Pollo performed a demonstrative study on the effects of verbally induced expectations on motor performance in patients with Parkinson's disease with implanted stimulating electrodes in the subthalamic nuclei.[5] After the stimulator had been turned off several times, with subsequent reductions in motor function, the participants were again told that the stimulator would be turned off. This time, however, the stimulator was left on at the normal basal rate. The verbal suggestion alone resulted in significant measurable reductions in the participant's motor function. This decrease was completely blocked when the opposite, positive verbal instructions were given, such as,"we will increase the intensity of the stimulator." This work is one of many that suggest that the specific words chosen by a physician, without any modifications to specific medications or procedures, may alter the outcome of a medical treatment.

The importance of a *patient's faith in the doctor and his or her prescribed treatment* has been recognized as a part of healing since

Hippocrates. Recommendations from trusted friends, information gleaned from newspapers, and important symbols such as the white coat and the framed diploma can all help to mold a patient's perception of the doctor's skill. In turn, these perceptions about the doctor can quickly build and alter the patient's beliefs about the treatment the clinician prescribes. Numerous studies have demonstrated the powerful effects that patients' belief in their doctor can have on the outcome of medical treatments. One interesting study by Hashish and Feinman did not set out to examine this topic, but ended up clearly demonstrating the clinical power of a "white coat."[6] The experiment set out to identify the most effective level of ultrasound therapy on pain reduction in patients who had recently undergone oral surgery. Surprisingly, the researchers found that the ultrasound therapy was an effective form of pain reduction even when the machine was turned off. The experimenters then hypothesized that the therapeutic effect was due to the massage of the injured area resulting from the application of the ultrasound apparatus. To test this hypothesis, they trained new patients to massage themselves with the inactive ultrasound head with the same movements used by the white coat-wearing professionals in the previous trials. Surprisingly, this new technique, despite being mechanically identical to the previous trials, was now completely ineffective. Evidently, the therapeutic benefit was not derived from the ultrasonic waves, or the massage, or the office, or even enrollment in the study; the therapeutic benefit was dependent upon the presence of a white coat-wearing professional. Without the involvement of the physician and everything he or she represented to the patient, the impressive therapeutic benefit of the treatment vanished.

A *patient's culture* is typically viewed only as a possible barrier to appropriate medical treatment. Currently most physicians in training are instructed to be alert to cultural interpretations as a potential hazard in patient encounters that can drive patients away from effective treatments. For example, cultural differences may make a routine physical exam seem insulting or prevent patients from understanding a doctor's instructions. Few physicians are taught about the significant positive effects a patient's culture can have on treatment outcomes.

Phillips and Ruth performed an unusual study examining whether a patient's culture was significantly affecting the most important clinical outcome of all: survival.[7] They examined the deaths of 28,169 Chinese Americans and nearly half a million randomly selected "white" (non-Asian) controls. They found that Chinese Americans, but not white Americans, died significantly earlier than normal (1.3 years compared to 4.9 years) if they had a combination of birth year and disease that Chinese philosophy and medical theories consider ill-fated. For example, Chinese Americans whose deaths were attributed to lymphatic cancer and who were born in "Earth years," who according to Chinese astrology are prone to develop illnesses with lumps, nodules, or tumors, had an average age of death of 59.7 years. Non-Chinese whites and Chinese Americans born during non-Earth years, however, had an average age of death that was nearly four years later (63.6 years) when diagnosed with lymphatic cancer. The intensity of this effect was found to directly correlate with the personal identification and commitment to traditional Chinese culture. Phillips and Ruth found that this held true for nearly all causes of death studied and could not be completely explained by changes in the behavior of the Chinese patient or the doctors involved. It seems that when the patients received a diagnosis related to their birth year, it validated and enhanced their culturally based beliefs and expectations, resulting in significant clinical detriment.

Lastly, over the past few years there has been growing support for the idea that what is widely known as the placebo effect is at least partially the result of *patient conditioning*. Rather than salivating like Pavlov's dogs, patients are said to respond to cues in the medical environment by initiating physiological processes necessary for healing. Patients with regular access to health care develop a life-long pattern of feeling ill, going to a doctor, taking a medication, and then feeling better. This pattern is then faithfully repeated, even if the medicine is not the specific source of the healing.

A series of clever experiments by Voudouris and colleagues demonstrated the effect of a conditioning experience on the participant's perception of pain.[8] The participants in this study were given a rising intensity of electric shocks, each noted with an audible clicking noise, and the current was established at which the shocks became painful and intolerable. The participants were then given an inert cream described as a powerful anesthetic and the shock trial was repeated. A fraction of the subjects demonstrated a placebo response by tolerating pain at higher intensities. Once this baseline "placebo rate" was established, the trial was run again with a new set of participants. During this new trial, however, after the inert cream was administered the strength of the electric shocks was turned down. The patient, unaware of any change in the machine's strength, now had the opportunity to observe the "effectiveness" of the inert cream. When more of the cream was applied and the trial was repeated, this time with the shock strength at the baseline level, larger numbers of the subjects (much larger than the original placebo rate) were able to endure higher-intensity shocks before they reported pain and intolerable pain. It seems that the conditioning trial with the inert cream and the experience of lower-strength electric shocks had a powerful effect on how the participants experienced pain.

The factors within the context of the patient–doctor encounter perform the unifying function of creating an expectation within the mind of the patient. Patients' past experiences, their culture, and all that they have heard and read about treatment and the doctor all come together to help them form an expectation about the treatment's outcome. Well-known clinical treatments, as well as placebos, seem to work significantly better when a patient is given the opportunity, and

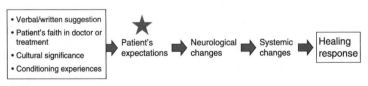

Figure 6.2

sometimes the guidance, to form positive expectations about the treatment. The previously discussed postoperative anesthesia trial by Benedetti and Colloca is a good example of how a patient's expectation can alter clinical outcomes. In that trial, patients who were shown the injection and given the information (i.e., "you are receiving a pain-relieving intervention") necessary to form an expectation required less pain medication and reported pain relief at a much faster rate than participants who received pain medicine from a hidden infusion pump. Research has shown a significant and replicable correlation between the degree of *expected success* of treatment and the clinical effectiveness of a treatment.[9]

Numerous researchers agree that a patient's expectations may be the psychological basis for the placebo response, or what we prefer to call the healing response. An expectation is not an imaginary, philosophical entity in the minds of patients. Neuroscience has shown that an expectation has an identifiable neurological counterpart. Expectations are correlated with a measurable change in the brain. Regions of the prefrontal cortex, specifically the dorsolateral aspect (DLPFC), are thought to maintain internal representations of goals and expectations, which then modify activity in other regions of the brain.[10]

Researchers recently added weight to this hypothesis when they found that activity in the DLPFC directly correlated with the magnitude of analgesia expected from a placebo administration by participants in an experimental pain trial.[11] Other regions of the prefrontal cortex, known as the orbitofrontal cortex (OFC) and the rostral anterior cingulated cortex (rACC), have also been linked to the cognitive and emotional appraisals of physiological processes such as pain.[12]

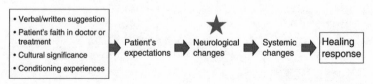

Figure 6.3

Neuronal activity within these three cerebral regions seems to be closely tied to the formation of a psychological expectation. A recent study examined activity in these regions during the anticipation period of a placebo analgesia experiment. Participants were scanned by functional magnetic resonance imaging (fMRI) as they received painful electric shocks to the wrist. After exposure to the electric shocks, some participants were given an "analgesic" cream. Participants were scanned as they waited variable amounts of time for the next electric shock. Researchers examined what brain activity the participants displayed during this time of expectation and found that the expectation of pain relief correlated with an increase in cerebral activity in the DLPFC, the OFC, and the rACC.[13] These findings were confirmed when another recent study found that the OFC, the rACC, and the DLPFC were all significantly more active in participants who had experienced a procedure designed to enhance expectations about an experimental outcome compared with those in the control group.[14]

Current evidence suggests that the presence of an expectation and the activation of the aforementioned areas of the cerebrum result in a "top-down" cascade where activity in the prefrontal cortex modulates activity in other areas of the cortex, in the subcortical nuclei, the midbrain, and eventually the brainstem. Numerous studies have confirmed that the formation of an expectation can affect the metabolic rate, the cerebral blood flow, and other general activity markers in other regions of the brain. One such study performed by Wager and Rilling examined how the expectation of pain relief affects the activity of pain-responsive regions of the brain: the thalamus, somatosensory cortex, insula, and anterior cingulate cortex. These areas of the brain show demonstrable increases in activity when a person experiences a painful stimulus.[15] Researchers hypothesized that if placebo manipulations were capable of mitigating the experience of pain, then the pain-responsive regions of the brain should show a correlating reduction in measures relating to neural activity. Participants were scanned with fMRI as they received painful electric shocks. After each shock participants were asked to rate the pain they experienced. fMRI scans of the shocks alone, without any placebo manipulations, revealed activation of the classic pain matrix: thalamus, somatosensory cortex/primary motor cortex, somatosensory cortex, anterior insula, anterior cingulate cortex, ventrolateral prefrontal cortex, and cerebellum. Some participants were then given an inert cream and were told it was a powerful analgesic, providing an expectation of pain relief. Another round of shocks confirmed that the self-reported pain was greater for control participants than those who had received the inert cream, indicating the formation of an analgesic expectation.

Significantly, researchers found that the magnitude of placebo analgesia reported by the participants correlated with a measurable reduction in neural activity in the pain-responsive regions of the brain. Wager and colleagues also noted that enhanced activity in the DLPFC, OFC, and rACC (regions associated with the formation of expectations) correlated with decreases in self-reported pain and decreases in activity in pain-associated regions of the brain.[16] The formation of an expectation was shown to directly correlate with changes in the neuronal activity of pain-related regions of the brain, as well as the personal experience of analgesia.

Another study found that a person's expectations were able to modulate the activity of neurons in the primary taste cortex, an area previously thought to respond solely to sensory input from taste receptors and lingual somatosensory receptors. Participants were exposed to a highly aversive bitter taste in two conditions, one where they were told truthfully that the taste was going to be very bitter and the other where they were led to believe that the taste was going to be far more pleasant than it actually was. When the participants formed positive expectations about the taste, the primary taste cortex demonstrated diminished activity (as measured with an fMRI scan) than when participants had an expectation of the foul taste.[17] Those participants who did not expect the bitter taste also self-reported the experience of a less bitter taste than those who had expected the foul taste. The primary taste cortex is not known to have any strong association with the DLPFC, rACC, or OFC, and yet

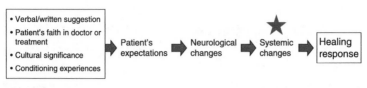

Figure 6.4

the introduction of expectation-induced modifications in these regions had a direct effect on the activity of the primary taste cortex.

It is becoming more and more clear that an expectation can affect neuronal activity in some, if not all, regions of the brain. The introduction or enhancement of a patient's expectation increases activity in the DLPFC, rACC, and OFC. These activated regions are then capable of modifying neuronal activity in other regions of the brain, even in the primary taste cortex.

In this "top-down" cerebral cascade, modifications in neuronal activity must eventually cumulate in alterations of physiological processes. Even if we do not fully understand the process, it is clear that modifications of cerebral activity have physiological consequences. Years of research in the area of placebo analgesia have generated a reasonably clear picture of how an expectation might do its work. Unlike the vast majority of placebo-related topics, placebo-induced analgesia has enjoyed decades of intense research. Since the 1970s, scientists have been building, piece by piece, a complete neurological and physiological story of how a placebo can result in a patient's pain relief. The mechanism behind placebo analgesia is not yet entirely understood. There are lingering questions and focal points of debate scattered throughout contemporary placebo research. In addition, the placebo effect, as we know it today, is likely the result not of a single mechanism but rather of multiple, intertwined complex mechanisms. The proposed mechanism behind some forms of placebo analgesia that we will discuss here serves as only an example of one of the many possibilities that may underlie this phenomenon.

The story of placebo analgesia begins with pain. All human beings are familiar with pain. It is a vital, although often unwelcome, sensation used to monitor the safety of our surroundings and our actions. The processing of a painful sensation takes place in an integrated matrix that spans the central and peripheral nervous systems. For the sake of discussion, we will use pain that originates in our body's periphery. Imagine that while cooking dinner a person accidentally places his hand on the hot stove, causing pain. As his skin hits the stove, receptors in the skin surface are activated, and two distinct populations of afferent axons, myelinated A delta fibers and unmyelinated C fibers, conduct the electrical impulse from the peripheral region to the spine. In the case of the hot stove, these fibers carry the pain sensation from the hand, up the arm, to the back, where they synapse in the substantia gelatinosa of the dorsal horn of the spinal cord. The famous "gate control" theory of pain processing, proposed and then further modified by Melzack and Wall, states that the neural input from the periphery to the dorsal horn effectively modulates the flow of impulses from the spinal cord to the brain.[18] In other words, not every neuronal signal from the hand is sufficient to generate a neuronal signal to the brain. It takes a certain number and magnitude of neuronal transmissions in the presence (or more importantly, the absence) of other competing neuronal signals to generate a successful signal to the brain. This point of flux, where different signals are integrated and balanced, is the "gate" the *sensation* of pain must pass through in order to become the cognitive *awareness* of pain. Only when stimulation from the periphery is sufficient will the sensation of pain be transmitted from the spinal cord to the thalamus and to the cerebral cortex, where it is processed and finally understood by the person to be "pain."

Activity in the brain can produce analgesia through descending inhibitory pathways that extend from the cortex down to this gate region of the spinal cord. We have already discussed how an expectation has the power to increase activity in areas of the cortex such as the DLPFC, OFC, and rACC. One of these regions, the rACC, has a direct connection to an important pain-processing region in the midbrain known as the periaqueductal gray. Converging evidence suggests that activity in the rACC stimulates an increase in activity in the periaqueductal gray by way of neuronal fiber tracts that directly link the two. Imaging studies that monitored brain activity during experiences of placebo-induced analgesia have confirmed that an increase in activity in the rACC covaries with an increase in activity in the periaqueductal gray.[19] Using rat models, Kandel and Schwartz and colleagues have demonstrated the importance of the periaqueductal gray in producing analgesia. Their experiment demonstrated that direct stimulation of the periaqueductal gray through injections of low-dose opiates results in profound systemic analgesia in the rat.[20] The periaqueductal gray then projects its neuronal fibers down to the nucleus raphe magnus in the medulla. Once the cascade of stimulation reaches the raphe magnus nucleus, fibers that extend from the medulla all the way down to the dorsal horn of the spinal cord are stimulated to release serotonin.

Recalling our earlier discussion of pain, we now return to the "gate." Fibers from the raphe magnus nucleus extend down and meet those pain fibers from the periphery in the substantia gelatinosa of the dorsal horn of the spinal cord. When activated, axons of the raphe magnus release serotonin into this crucial "gate" region and in doing so activate inhibitory interneurons. These interneurons are neurons that exist within the spinal cord to modify the chemical transmission between various synapses. When the axons of the raphe magnus release serotonin, the interneurons are stimulated to release their own bundles of neurotransmitters—which in this case happen to be endogenous opioids. The opioid molecules bind their matching receptor on the incoming peripheral pain axons and prevent those fibers from transmitting the pain signal up the spinal cord to the brain. The peripheral pain axons are silenced, and the pain message has officially been lost in transit.

We do not offer the biological schema developed here as *the* model, but as *a* model. It is one possible account of how something as simple as a clinician's words can result in pain relief. As research on the impact of mental states on physiology continues, the neurological pathways involved will be further elucidated. Today, however, there is more than enough clinical evidence that what a patient thinks, feels, and perceives truly matters, and that the effects of the skills we have described can be modeled in terms of what we know about neuroscience.

RETHINKING THE PLACEBO EFFECT AS THE HEALING RESPONSE

Traditionally, the studies we have described and numerous other studies of the therapeutic effects of clinician–patient relationships are categorized as "placebos" or "placebo effects." This is unfortunate since it masks their true importance. Placebos are typically defined as "inert," "inactive," or "nonspecific" interventions and frequently as ethically suspect or "sham medicine." In addition, the use of placebos as the standard against which new drugs are tested suggests that the power of placebos is recognized, but at the same time, a drug found to be "no better than placebo" is regarded as a failure. This is a legacy of medicine's impressive scientific gains and technological orientation, yet as Miller and Kaptchuk have argued, it is misleading as a way to conceptualize and adequately account for this important phenomenon.[21]

In fact, placebos are not inert, nor do they require a dummy pill or sham procedure to be effective. The active pharmacological agents in the placebo effect have been repeatedly shown to be endogenous opioids, dopamine release, and other agents for which the precise biological triggers and pathways have yet to be fully identified. Yet it is clear that patient expectations of being helped, cultural conditioning, and the quality of clinician–patient relationships are involved and can make a real difference in health outcomes. In light of this research, a major rethinking of placebos and placebo effects, and with it a new understanding of healing, is required.[22] This rethinking is still in its infancy and constitutes a major challenge for health practice and education.

In one sense the findings of researchers like Colloca, Kaptchuk, and Kiecolt-Glaser are not likely to be surprising to clinicians, who frequently see their patients get better because of positive reinforcement, the creation of a healing environment in their clinics and among their staff, and specific encouragement to patients about the likely benefits of interventions. Nor is it likely to surprise anyone who has been seen by a skilled practitioner and begun to feel better from the very beginning of the visit because of the way the relationship was established. Yet there has been little place for either the research findings or the intuitive wisdom of practitioners and patients until recently. And most schools of medicine, still working within a predominantly biomechanical model of health and illness, have yet to find a place for the emerging evidence for what has been widely described as the work of placebos, or what Miller and Kaptchuk understand as the power of context. They have put the issue well: "Instead of focusing exclusively on the therapeutic power of medical technology and thereby ignoring or dismissing context, we should see the context of the clinical encounter as a potential enhancer, and in some cases the primary vehicle, of therapeutic benefit." They conclude that future work "should aim at isolating and elucidating those factors in the clinician–patient encounter that contribute causally to improvement in outcomes for patients."[23] This is precisely the work we have begun to describe in this book.

We believe that the best way to describe the constellation of factors resulting in patient improvement involving placebos, contextual factors, expectations, and the cascade of physiological changes is "the healing response." This phrase focuses appropriately on the relational dimension of what is experienced—that it is a response of the patient. It also highlights that the most important thing about this constellation of phenomena is that the patient benefits. It leaves open questions of just how these benefits occur, encouraging further research, while freeing us from the more pejorative connotations of "placebos" or "placebo effect" and the impersonal connotations associated with terms like "context."

Throughout the book we have used the term "healing" in its customary, everyday usage to discuss a wide range of human experiences, as reported by our practitioners. In this chapter we have been examining a more limited domain that we are calling "the healing response."

More precisely, we have argued for this phrase as a replacement for "placebo effect." "Healing" is the larger category, "healing response" the smaller one, referring to those parts of the larger domain that have been studied within the scientific paradigm. We do not assume that the scientific paradigm will provide an adequate means to study all instances of healing.

The idea that relationships matter in patient healing and that these relationships also affect practitioner well-being is given additional importance by recent research on the brain. Some of the most exciting recent work in neuroscience indicates that relational skills can be learned and improved throughout life. Over the past two decades neuroscientist Richard Davidson has produced a body of research findings strongly suggesting that the brain is more changeable than previously thought, even during adulthood.[24] By mapping neural activity in people during a wide range of activities, Davidson has substantially advanced our understanding of the interactivity between emotional states, brain activity, and a range of human skills and abilities. For example, the "brain maps" of technicians who practiced meditation for only three hours per week showed increased activity in the left prefrontal cortex, the main area responsible for positive emotions. Davidson's studies are one example of a growing body of research that indicates a human capacity to shape and recalibrate emotional makeup, and the range of human skills that are tied to emotional well-being.

These insights are at least as old as the Buddha's teachings that people have some power to control their thoughts and emotions, and thereby alter their lives, through mindfulness. One prominent health-related application of the healing power of mindfulness is the work of Jon Kabat-Zinn at the Mindfulness-Based Stress Reduction (MBSR) Clinic at the University of Massachusetts Medical Center. The research of Kabat-Zinn with Davidson and their colleagues has demonstrated that MBSR could reduce the subjective sense of suffering, improve immune function, and speed healing. Most important for our focus here, they showed that MBSR was beneficial for interpersonal relationships and improved patients' general sense of well-being.[25] Harnessing these findings for better education in the health professions and better healthcare practices is the challenge that lies ahead. We will turn to this task in the next section.

To summarize: Our interviews indicate that many practitioners may have a keen awareness of the power of relationships, yet confirming biomedical studies have not been available until relatively recently. What is new is the amount of neuroscience research establishing the connections between brain structures and well-being, and strong indications that the quality of practitioner–patient relationships is important to healing. More precisely, what is genuinely novel in this field could be summarized as three things: (1) the ability to see through SPECT (single proton emission computerized tomography) and fMRI (functional magnetic resonance imaging) the biochemical changes in the brain that correspond to various emotional, stressed, or relaxed states; (2) a growing awareness that those mental/emotional states, which are crucial to effective relationships, can be learned and relearned; and (3) a developing knowledge of which relational skills produce positive patient outcomes and a better understanding of their biochemical pathways.

TOWARD A NEW PARADIGM FOR EDUCATION IN MEDICINE

Some may see the research we have reviewed in this chapter as new and promising, while for others these studies may simply confirm their clinical experience. The general understanding that the practitioner's capacity for compassionate relationships is a key component in healing is as old as Western medicine itself and has been embodied in the experience of expert practitioners for millennia. The Hippocratic tradition encouraged the use of humanism in order to truly "heal" a patient, which even in ancient Greece meant more than "curing" his or her disease. "The patient, though conscious that his condition is perilous, may recover his health simply through his contentment with the goodness of the physician."[26]

Since the Flexner Report of 1910, U.S. medical schools have become extremely adept at teaching therapeutic interventions at the biological level, but much less adept at teaching the other skills that contribute to health—communication, the establishment of trusting relationships, attention to the cultural significance of illness, and especially the compassionate use of physicians' considerable powers to influence their patients' well-being beyond mechanically fixing the body. There is a growing sense nationally that exclusive reliance on the paradigm of the Flexner Report, with its narrow focus on biological functions, no longer serves us well. It perpetuates an incomplete model for medicine and needs to be incorporated into a larger vision, shaped by the best research on what makes people well and keeps them well. Ironically, several scholars have claimed that Flexner himself was unhappy that his report had resulted in a fixation on the sciences to the exclusion of broader issues of the meaning of doctoring that can be learned through studies in the humanities. As Rabow and colleagues put it in a recent report in *Academic Medicine*, "We now have an opportunity to pick up all the threads of Flexner's work and reweave into our professional education an emphasis on personal integrity, moral character and service values."[27] Our thesis in this volume takes a step further. By paying attention to recent studies of the profound importance of relational factors in healing, we have an opportunity to develop a new paradigm for medicine, integrating the best of the basic sciences with humanistic skills. What is at stake is not only the professionalism of the doctor as a service provider, but also the quality of care patients receive. Humanistic skills, such as the ones we describe in this volume, turn out to be important not only to the doctor's moral identity but also to his or her ability to help patients get better.

The 1994 Pew-Fetzer Task Force Report on "Health Professions Education and Relationship-Centered Care" is one landmark in the recognition of the need for a new medical model.[28] More recently, the Institute of Medicine's (IOM) 2001 report "Crossing the Quality Chasm" said that care based on "continuous healing relationships" is the key to redesigning the system.[29] These are encouraging signs that a new paradigm is in the process of taking hold. We hope this volume will lend additional weight to this effort.

We have been concerned here with summarizing what we think is a representative body of the important recent research on the neuroscience of healing. Understanding that there is scientific backing behind this renewed call for healing relationships, and not simply idealistic rhetoric, gives the educational and organizational reforms described by the Pew-Fetzer Task Force and the IOM more weight and urgency. In brief, clinician–patient relationships are more central to the healing process than the current biomechanical understanding of human illness acknowledges.[30] Doctors and other health professionals can no longer be concerned simply with knowledge and skills that facilitate *technical competence*, but must acquire skills such as empathy, compassion, and agility in communication that lead to *relational competence*, which in turn promotes and facilitates healing.

This has major implications for medical education in particular. Novack and colleagues correctly note that relational skills are usually considered "soft," and the educational opportunities concerned with such skills are seen as less valuable and are often optional rather than required experiences.[31] Therefore, we should not be surprised that medical graduates, while very bright and full of information, are sometimes ill equipped for effective patient care. The challenge before us is one of re-imagining medical education as preparing physicians to be healers, as well as to cure acute diseases and manage chronic ones. One essential part of this re-imagining lies in understanding that the future quality of patient care is vitally linked to medical students' self-awareness, personal growth, and well-being. Caring well for others is grounded in caring well for oneself, as our next chapter on self-care will amply illustrate. Daniel Siegel summarizes the importance of compassionate self-awareness in his book *The Mindful Brain*. Noting the way that studies have linked good interpersonal relationships with health, Siegel proposes that "mindful awareness is a form of self-relationship, an internal form of attunement that creates similar states of health."[32] This applies to both health professionals and the patients for whom they care. Promoting and nurturing such mindful self-awareness should be a major agenda for medical and healthcare education at all levels.

In short, the current dominant model of medical education does not provide adequate opportunity for students to develop relational skills, and it fosters too little in the areas of self-awareness and personal growth, which are prerequisites for practicing these skills. More work is needed to ensure that health professions students understand how their personal attitudes and emotions, their biases, and their relational skills (or lack of them) can substantially affect their clinical abilities. Sharon Dobie puts it well when she indicates how significant a change this would be, and she calls for "a paradigm shift to a culture where teachers and learners are willing to consciously attend to their relationships and to the work on self-awareness and mindfulness while they also master the biomedical knowledge required of the profession."[33]

We have worked so long in the shadow of the Flexner Report and the valorization of the basic biological sciences as the only essential elements of medical education that what Dobie and others recommend regarding relational awareness and self-reflection has often been thought of as a desirable "add-on," but not a feature of the core curriculum. For 100 years the accepted wisdom has been that humane characteristics are fine so long as physicians are first certified as technically competent. The recent findings of neuroscience show this to be an impoverished view, a dualism that separates cognition from feeling, competence as a technical skill from compassionate communication, and the analytical mind from the moral sensibilities. Our interviews have shown this to be operational nonsense. It is also educational nonsense. Recent research in the neurosciences supports the experiential wisdom of skilled clinicians. A 21st-century approach to health science education will incorporate all that we now understand from both the quantitative and qualitative sciences to train practitioners who will understand the healing potential of relationships and gain skill in wielding this impressive power. We end with a few suggestions aimed at medical and other health professions educators.

NOTES FOR EDUCATORS

1. Think of medical education as tending a garden rather than running a factory.
2. Think of students as organic, growing, whole persons, whose experiences in the educational process will either enhance or diminish their ability to help their patients.
3. Pay careful attention to the degree and kind of self-knowledge students acquire while becoming professionals. Too often medical education is an exercise in delayed maturation, which breeds resentment and the need for material rewards to compensate for the emotionally stunting features of their training. This makes it less likely that they can prize relational skills in themselves, or relate well to their patients.
4. Teach students to cultivate their own well-being. Teach the value of mindfulness and reflection, and the importance of exercise and good nutrition. Keep them in touch with whatever is sacred and beautiful in their lives. If they are not healthy themselves they cannot help others to heal. Faculty must of course model this, or it will become just another item on the impersonal checklist of "professionalism."
5. Provide students ample opportunity to reflect on what things provide them with meaning and support. This will increase their capacity for empathy with the meaning and support structures their patients bring to the clinic.
6. Teach the neuroscience of healing together with opportunities to practice and improve the relational skills involved in healing. Stress that this is evidence-based, cognitive-emotional work, not idealistic fluff.
7. Build a developmentally appropriate curriculum for all stages of professional education. Healing skills are both life skills, things one needs to survive and flourish, and lifetime skills, things that will mature over decades in practice.

[7]

HEALING THYSELF: CLINICIANS TALK ABOUT THEIR OWN HEALING PRACTICES

Listen carefully. As patient, as doctor, as health professional, as human being. It might just save your life.

—Jon Kabat-Zinn

In previous chapters we have been concerned with the wide range of ways that physicians facilitate healing in their patients. We now turn our focus to practitioners and how they attend to their own health and healing. We asked each of the 50 expert clinicians we interviewed a variation of this question: "What activities that promote wellness, wholeness, and healing do you personally engage in?" This chapter explores the responses we received to this question.

We begin with an interview that speaks to a wide range of both sufferings and self-care practices, remarkable for its courage and candor.

I: Could you talk about some of the things you do to sustain your own sense of health and wholeness?

P: I'm the right one to talk to about this; after 27 years of dealing with the sick and dying, believe me, I am horrifically burned out. I do everything in the world to keep myself propped up, to keep going for another year, and another year and another year. And I keep saying I'm going to do this one or two more years and then get completely out of it. I've been saying that for over five years.

I: So something is keeping you going.

P: I am being propped up; I don't know how healthy it is. Sometimes I think it's my liberation theology point of view. You know, I've tried everything.

From this more wholesale assessment, the practitioner then spoke of particular practices that have been helpful.

P: I went to the mind–body thing and learned their techniques. I spent four weeks on the West Coast in the "Death Workshops." They weren't called that, they were called something real cognitive— doctors won't go unless you've got a cognitive label on it, because everything has to be up in your head. But they were ways to let people get their feelings out.

I: Right.

P: I try to exercise, but I don't exercise as much as I need to. That's the hard part . . . sometimes things that are the simplest are the answer. You can learn all kinds of expensive stress management stuff, and there are all kinds of holistic people. Sometimes, the simplest things are right in front of you.

I: Yes.

P: I try to do things that give me joy and happiness. Going to the gym and working the weights does not give me joy and happiness. I've always said, "The final, common pathway to health is through joy." My coffee is good for me, because it is so full of joy. My chocolate that I eat every single day is good for me, because it is so full of joy. I think the final, common pathway is joy. And also, the physical activity that helps me the most is walking out in nature, hiking. And that's just essential. Was it Thoreau who said that there isn't a man who can be depressed in nature? Well, that's oversimplistic, but there's something to it. I have tried yoga. Yoga is my second choice, but it's hard to get to and expensive. I wish they had yoga right here in the hospital every morning, and

I could just walk in the door and go to yoga, and then go upstairs. That would be perfect. Doesn't happen. We don't do what we need to do in health care. So I love yoga . . . and something that has really healed me to a great degree is knitting. And the simplest things are so profound sometimes. You can be still and knit. You can be mentally still and knit. . . . It's just the brain in neutral. I love it. Hours a day sometimes. It's truly healed me.

Then the clinician ends with an overall assessment, rejecting standard psychiatric categories in favor of the larger assessment of the meaning of the suffering.

P: What's happened to me since then is that I'm not as happy a person. . . . I see the world as a darker place. And some people say, "You're depressed." I'm not depressed. Depression is about me. I don't feel bad about me. I feel like I'm OK. I feel bad about the sadness of the world, that I see the sadness more and more. It just breaks your heart more, and I know I was medicating a lot of that away. You know, that is there all the time. The world is a hard and sad place. Bad things happen; people suffer.

I: It's a tough world.

P: And a lot of people medicate themselves, one way or another; food or drinking or whatever. There's so many ways. So I have a little more—I tell my husband, "It's not depression; it's grief." I'm grieving the world. Grieving the world.

We do not enter this terrain of self-care lightly. Practitioners suffer, just as their patients suffer. Few other occupations place the service providers in the path of such a constant flow of pain and anxiety. Few other professionals engage in work in which the help they offer must be mediated and negotiated with the sufferer, and require the active assistance of the person being helped. Police officers and firemen sometimes save people from harm or death, and at personal risk, but these rescues usually occur without existential engagement with the social histories and personal idiosyncrasies of those being assisted. Except in emergency room rescues in which the patient is unconscious, health professionals have to go through—and with—their patients in order to help them. This can and does take a toll.

Moreover, expectations from patients and their families are often unrealistically high. In part this is a reflection of the neediness and vulnerability that comes with sickness. In part it is a function of the near-mythic curative expectations that American culture has placed on modern biomedical science. A culture that has been taught to turn to medical science for its salvation may have less tolerance for suffering and limitations on the alleviation of suffering. This adds to the practitioner's burden and makes practitioners' self-care all the more important.

Yet while the burdens of caregiving may be special, the skills of self-care for practitioners may not be. Health practitioners, like all of us, often keep themselves balanced, whole, and healthy through what the practitioner quoted above called "the simplest things"—through a strong family life, dedicated time with spouses and children, friendships with colleagues and in the community, exercises like running or Tai Chi, meditative practices like yoga or Qi Gong, and spiritual exercises like walking in the woods or attending religious services. The practitioners we interviewed discussed all these common self-care strategies. Yet because health practice is distinctive if not unique in its demands, we should expect to find special features to clinicians' self-care rituals and distinctive occasions for their performance. Hence as we describe some of the more common practices used for personal restoration, we will keep an eye focused on the particular forms these restorative practices take for healthcare practitioners.

Our assumption throughout is that clinicians themselves must have recovery, renewal, and healing if they are to carry the burden of caring for the sick. Attending to others depends, we assume, on some regular attention being given to oneself. In this way routine self-care and good patient care are critically interdependent.

SELF-CARE: SOME BASIC STRATEGIES

The term "basic" calls for some unpacking. By basic we do not mean elementary or simple, something for beginners. Indeed, our practitioners were largely well seasoned in self-care, the very opposite of novices. The strategies for self-care we discuss here are "basic" in the sense of foundational or supportive, necessary elements or building blocks at the base of health and wholeness. Failure to master some form of these self-care strategies would undermine healing capacities.

Creating Boundaries and Compartmentalizing

Patients, and often their families, carry with them to the clinic and into the hospital a variety of burdens, many of them nonmedical. As patients we never leave our baggage at the door. How could we? We are people, and our illnesses occur within the narrative structures that give coherence and meaning to our lives. We want to be recognized for who we are, especially perhaps when we are sick and our fundamental sense of self is damaged or compromised. As Anatole Broyard says, we all want the doctor to come to our illnesses through our personality.[1] This was described vividly in the chapter on patient perceptions of the doctor–patient interaction. And of course this can be a source of enormous intrinsic rewards for the practitioner, but also a major burden of the work.

One of the most basic fears of practitioners is being swallowed up in the hurt and suffering that patients present. If they empathize with each patient, if they get to know each patient's larger life narrative and become an empathic witness to each patient's wounded humanity, they just might be overwhelmed by it. Psychiatrist Jodi Halpern puts it vividly in describing the effort to maintain what she calls "emotional homeostasis": "Doctors continually deal with issues people dislike viewing realistically—death, dying, suffering and loss." Because of this, perhaps, taking a hyperrational approach to one's emotional involvement is a way of buffering oneself, "to protect ourselves from harsh reality."[2]

The consistent message of our expert healers is that this fear is present and powerful, but the tactic of emotional distancing is often counterproductive. Not to take seriously the affective valences of care is to forego much of the healing potential of relationships. One clinician describes the consequence of too much armor as beginning to think of patients as "it," or as "not us." Unless clinicians can listen and provide some empathic presence, they will know less about their patients and they will be less effective in providing guidance. Our expert clinicians know very well that being open to patients is an important part of healing them, but that it also can be costly. So part of self-care lies in the ability to hear the suffering and to empathize, but not be threatened or overwhelmed by it.

One clinician who works with children talked about this in some detail. He described what occurs when parents approach the clinician saying, "My child is bad," out of bounds, and acting out all the time. It helps, he said, to separate the illness from the behavior. For example, if the immediate problem is out-of-bounds behavior but the illness behind it is posttraumatic stress disorder, focusing on the diagnosis, which can then become the focus of therapy, is a helpful strategy. "If I look only at the behavior or the environment I am going to be overwhelmed." So an interest in the disease itself, bracketing for a while the behavioral and environmental problems, is a way of caring for oneself, as well as a useful reorientation for the child and the parents.

Halpern discusses this tactic and illustrates it using both ancient and modern sources. Being strategic about emotions, educating the emotions to seek a focus on the long-term interests of others, rather than the short-term and often disturbing reactions that situations evoke in us, is as old as Aristotle. And Buddhists have developed a variety of meditation practices for nearly 2,500 years designed to offer release from the tyranny of emotions, while developing compassion. Many of our clinicians practiced some process of selective emotional attentiveness. Studies of various styles of practitioner–patient relationships by Roter and colleagues add some empirical validation to these practices. In Roter's studies the highest physician satisfaction is associated with practitioners who have good emotional communication with their patients, rather than those whose style is emotionally restricted and more narrowly bioscientific.[3]

Another instance of boundary creation and bracketing involves dealing with the grief that is caused when patients don't get better, or get worse. Some patients continue to suffer or die despite the clinician's best efforts. Here a strategy some clinicians discussed involves a recognition that no one can be, nor should anyone try to be, immune to the human tragedy that is sometimes presented.

> I do have the ability to compartmentalize. When I was in pediatric cardiology I was dealing with kids with congenital heart problems, and of course I would become quite fond of these kids, and not uncommonly, they'd have terrible things happen and die. And I had to learn how not to be so devastated that I couldn't keep going on, to be effective for other people, and so, the way I learned subconsciously to deal with that is to allow myself to have a bit of grief, but then to compartmentalize it. I mean you never really lose the grief, but, somehow, you put it over here [gesturing to the side].

This testament of learning to honor one's grief without being disabled or overcome by it is at the core of self-care. "What to do with the grief" was a recurring theme. The effort to shut it out completely with denial, self-medication, or failure to engage with patients was viewed as not only detrimental to patients, but a self-destructive response.

This same practitioner then deepened his story by identifying how honoring and then compartmentalizing his grief allowed him to focus on the present. This echoes the emphasis in Chapter 1 on giving undistracted attention to patients. He continued: "But I've become operationally fairly existential, and I developed a philosophy that fundamentally we deal in the here and now, and the world around us, in our attempt to do what we can do to improve it. So that's how I am able to put [aside] some of those things that in my youth would have incapacitated me."

Then this quick self-assessment: "I hope I haven't become inured, lost sensitivity. Actually, I haven't become inured, in that I still have the same kind of pain; it's just that I'm able to live with it."

Although none of our clinicians discussed the issues of emotional engagement or disengagement with patients in terms of a formal model, their comments were akin to Halpern's model of clinical empathy and emotional reasoning. Her model rejects the two common models of empathy: "detached concern," which is care that distances the practitioner from the patient, and "affective merging," in which the clinician becomes one with the patient's suffering. In Halpern's paradigm, practitioners should seek "to resonate emotionally with, yet stay aware of, what is distinctive about the patient's experience."[4] In her view this is done through a kind of imaginative attunement, in which clinicians stay open to the hints and gestures that patients give for things not on the clinician's checklist or routine stock of questions—and then put these to therapeutic use. Obvious examples are patient tears or nervous silences in response to a clinician's questions, but more subtle changes in tone and inflection of voice or body postures can also be important. Halpern continues: "When physicians meet these hints with detached responses, no disclosure takes place." In contrast, when clinicians attend to these hints and gestures, patients often discuss more emotionally charged areas and provide better histories.[5] Halpern concludes: "The pursuit of a correct diagnosis requires a full, as well as accurate understanding of the patient's problems," and then a therapeutic interaction becomes possible.[6]

Staying Aware

Another basic self-care practice was awareness. One practitioner gave us this description:

> I take at least two minutes between each patient. . . . I check in with myself. Am I OK? Am I now ready to hear another story? If I'm not OK, I will clear my head, listen to a little music, burn a little

incense, perhaps write a few e-mails. It's worth being a few minutes late to be fully present to that person.

A family practitioner used a similar kind of refocusing, but more selectively.

I know if I have a complex patient to see I just say this quick prayer: I don't have the insight into human nature that you [God] do, not at all, but you do. Just give me a key for what they need. Help me understand them well enough and love them well enough that I can understand what they really need.

This practitioner explained this prayer practice as "preparation of my own mind," as a way of approaching patients without the need to find a quick answer, without a sense of urgency, or to avoid rushing the patient through the visit. So it would be a mistake to interpret this as a form of intercessory prayer, in which the clinician is asking for a divine intervention or revelation. It is better described as a reverent self-exhortation for giving the next patient full attention. Clearly the clinician's intention is to create an opening in which things could unfold or develop in a way that would disclose the real problem, or the problem for which the clinician might have a response or remedy. We discussed this motif earlier in terms of making and holding a space in which the healing can develop, with the recognition that giving time and attention is a key. This clinician's prayer is essentially a request for an undivided attention, a clear focus on the patient in the here and now.

While some practitioners took time between each patient or before seeing patients with complex problems, other practitioners started their day with the recitation of life guides—short wisdom sayings or maxims that helped them become oriented for the day's work. The most comprehensive list of such guides was given to us by a former emergency physician who, because of a career-limiting injury, had turned his skills to a practice requiring fewer acute and more chronic care skills. His list of guides was remarkable in its eclecticism, drawing from a wide range of philosophical, psychological, and spiritual traditions. The one guide he discussed in detail was a pledge to enact an attitude of unconditional positive regard. "I will bring to each encounter an unconditional positive regard to bring out the compassion, forgiveness, love, and healing in each of us." The phrase "unconditional positive regard," as this practitioner understood it, was taken from Buddhist *metta* meditation practices, the offering of loving-kindness to the universe and all beings in it. This practice carries with it the idea that such intention and blessing open the gateway to "compassion, forgiveness, love, and healing." Interestingly, also included in this clinician's life-guide list was a separate maxim focusing directly on forgiveness, not as a product of unconditional positive regard, but as a skill or capacity in its own right. Forgiveness may be called for in such practice when a transgression needs to be recognized and released, even when unconditional positive regard is present. For example, situations involving child or spousal abuse may call for separate acts of forgiveness, whether the patient is the transgressor or the victim. Combining the practice of unconditional positive regard with forgiveness provides opportunities for cultivating deeper awareness of self and others.

The life guides point to and can be part of another basic self-care practice: self-awareness. One clinician put it this way:

This is not about me, not about me. It is not even about death. It is about being big—being, just not doing—but being. There's a quote I heard years ago: "The most influential part of the healing of the patient is the consciousness of the doctor." And I believe that. When I am healthy and in tune and balance myself I believe that to be true.

The "consciousness" of clinicians, in the sense it is used here, is developed by cultivating their own self-awareness, the range and depth of what they are able to attend to outside themselves. When they are not centered and in touch with their best self, their most aware self, then "I do all the right things mechanically, but it's a different experience."

When "in tune" with themselves, however, "it's powerful to people, and I have more energy at the end of the day than when I started."

Central to this idea of cultivating one's own self-awareness is the importance of sustaining a practice—that is, of it being done *daily*. As the term implies, a practice is a repeated, embodied activity, not simply a cerebral affirmation of a set of principles. Practice is necessary for developing proficiency, whether it is a professional practice or a personal one. The idea that healers recognize a need for a consistently engaged, self-care practice alongside their professional practice is a theme we will return to later. For now we simply wish to note the idea, consistently stressed in the interviews, that a practice has to be routinely enacted and concretely felt to have useful long-term effects. As emphasized in the interview that opens this chapter, practitioners may need a cognitive label for a self-care practice because it first has to be "up in their heads." But the actual value of the self-care practice becomes more bodily, not through thinking it but through doing it. The practitioner with the list of life guides put it this way: "I go for it because it works. Over time I can notice when one [of the life guides] begins to creep into my life, as a reference point for decisions."

Practicing a Full Life

Another powerful and basic self-care strategy we learned from our informants could be called simply living a full life. One practitioner talked about working on his farm as opening a full range of engagement in life. And he said that he found the lessons he learned there were more valuable than continuing medical education: "Spending time having a vital life is more important than reading medical journals." One example: "Things die on the farm—but we go on."

Another practitioner talked about playing the guitar and the piano, and being aware of herself in those capacities. She made an explicit connection between experiencing herself in these activities and recognizing multiple dimensions of her patients: "There is so much more to their story because I know there is so much more to my story. I help [my patients] connect with all of themselves rather than the small story [about their diabetes or depression] that someone fed them."

To our expert clinicians a full life often meant taking enough time away from the office or hospital, time with spouses and children or time for oneself alone. But this was not described as merely time "put in" for these activities. It was typically discussed as time devoted to *practicing* these activities, just as one practices medicine or health care—engaging in them routinely and self-consciously. "We have to practice life, and not just practice medicine," one clinician said. "There is a routine to it." One does it every day; there is a rhythm, a pulse or tempo to it. The same practitioner spoke of his practice of developing stillness in himself. Doing it daily, "like Roger Federer practicing his backhand," creates a "rhythm that pervades whatever you do." "If you don't do the practice of allowing the rhythm to develop in you, then you never get to the point of allowing that to happen with the things that you do in the real world."

COMMON BARRIERS AND HOW PRACTITIONERS OVERCOME THEM

But of course, exercising skills of self-care is no simple matter. Practitioners also spoke at length about some of the barriers to self-care, which occasionally involved lack of recognition of just how important self-renewal practices are. Sometimes it was simply a matter of not taking enough time for themselves. Indeed, many of the practitioners we interviewed talked ruefully about their own inadequacies or inconsistencies in self-care. So perhaps even aware-ness of the importance of attending to their own wholeness is not enough—until they find that lack of self-care is a major pitfall that reduces the quality of life for themselves and also leads to inferior patient care.

Every Waking Hour

One of our interviewees began this part of the discussion with an exclamation: "The struggle to maintain sanity!" Medical practitioners do have a threat to their sanity that is far above average, as evinced by the high rates of depression, suicide, and burnout among practitioners, as well as the variety of maladaptive coping strategies, such as alcohol abuse and drug use. This same clinician had sorted out his personal struggle by framing it as a question, "To whom is the physician primarily responsible?" And his answer was, "You're primarily responsible to yourself." He continued, "The old paradigm was that medicine was a jealous and demanding mistress, that it is a privilege to practice medicine, and that you can never fully know the art and science of that, and so it demands your every waking hour . . . and if you make that sacrifice then you can approach greatness in the profession." Many of the physicians that we interviewed heard this message early in their education and had it reiterated consistently throughout their training. But this clinician, like many, now recognized that the downside of this singular devotion was catastrophic: "And that [training] produced a lot of very smart, very good physicians whose spouses divorced them and whose kids hated them."

One practitioner spoke poignantly about a broken first marriage that had been "sacrificed on the altar of achievement." He continued, "I put my career much too far ahead of other commitments at that time and ended up paying for it." His second marriage and his practice have been successful in his view because "she doesn't give me any slack. She calls it like it is, and it is just immensely helpful."

One solution was to reinvent the formula for being a good clinician. "I think the paradigm that is more appropriate is that to be a good doctor you have to be a good human being, and to be a good human being you have to have a balanced life." The balance for this primary care clinician came through attending to his spiritual life, and being clear about those relationships that were most important to him and then nurturing them, finding "time to play" and "time to take care of yourself."

Because he tended to be an introvert, this clinician knew he needed quiet time to himself, and so his second struggle was with what he called "the disease of busyness." Being constantly accessible to patients, patients' families, and colleagues was a familiar feature to many we interviewed. In addition to land lines, faxes, and pagers, there are now e-mails and cell phones, all bringing to the clinician a cacophony of obligations. The "jealous and demanding mistress" has many helpers, all covetous of the practitioner's time and energy, all claiming importance and often urgency. Coming to the realization that one is primarily responsible to oneself helped one clinician to lower, if not entirely eliminate, this barrier to self-care.

The Practitioner as Martyr

A related barrier to self-care is the need to be important, and to feel oneself as important, perhaps even indispensable. One clinician, describing how much time he had spent on his practice earlier in his life, put it in these words: "A lot of my availability was because I felt an obligation to be there, to be the one, to be on call, to be available, to be this wonderful, self-sacrificing, dedicated physician. I felt so important, so valuable, and valued." This practitioner now sees this "high" of self-importance as "dangerous." Many clinicians, perhaps, have a strong need to be seen an invaluable, indispensable, the person without whom things would fall apart, or at least in whose absence things would go less well.

This physician now believes he was lucky to have had some good friends and a series of circumstances "to knock my ego down a notch or two. This was very helpful. So I don't have preconceived notions of my own self-importance anymore." Interestingly, the more positive paradigm came to this clinician from the world of music, when he heard a musician talk in glowing terms not of his own work but about the talent of others he had discovered, and how he began to understand his role as bringing in and nurturing talent that exceeded his own. This clinician subsequently began bringing partners into his practice that embodied his principles but who "would do better than I would."

The idea that no one can do it quite as well as I can, that the whole world depends on me to get it right, and that I should sacrifice myself to the great mission of caring for the sick, is, of course, not only delusional but a recipe for burnout. Most of our expert clinicians reported having learned, sometimes painfully, that "the world will go on without each of us."

But even in the absence of an exaggerated self-importance there is a temptation to be inordinately attached to the work, because health care always concerns people in need, sometimes great need. It would be simple and effortless to find oneself captivated by the importance of one's job. One practitioner put it succinctly: "It would be very easy never to let go of the work." Ironically, those physicians who have the best kinds of interactions with their patients may be precisely those who are most tempted to disregard themselves and give themselves body and soul to their practices. Yet for the clinicians we interviewed there was often another voice that warned of the problems of this singular dedication. Sometimes that voice was that of a family member. One clinician who finds escape and recuperation in exercise and reading said this: "My husband every once in a while will come home with a book and hand it to me"—a signal that the clinician was showing stress and needed some rebalancing. More than a few times in our interviews the voice of self-care that preserved or restored balance turned out to be the voice of the spouse or partner.

THE DIALECTIC OF HEALING

Earlier we alluded to a pervasive theme in the interviews concerning the way self-care is intimately tied to how one cares for patients. We now want to explore that theme in greater detail. Writer Anatole Broyard has described the dialectic of patient care and self-care in this way: "Not every patient can be saved, but his illness may be eased by the way the doctor responds to him—and in responding to him the doctor may save himself."[7]

Our clinician informants seemed well aware of this reciprocity of healing. One practitioner said it directly:

> What I find for the most part is that I get good energy from the people who come here, so I hope there is some mutual transfer of energy, because on the one hand, I may help people, that is possible. But the other side of it is my being enhanced by the people who come to see me. . . . I don't want to sound like I'm using my practice, but inadvertently, I do use my patients. I use them in the sense that they are my healing.

In a similar way, a remarkably large portion of our interviewees noted that patient encounters, and patients themselves, were often a source of renewal and healing for them. This should not be surprising. Given the long hours most clinicians devote to their practice, if the sources of renewal were completely outside the work, the burnout rate would undoubtedly be higher. Finding renewal as an intrinsic quality of the healthcare practice, getting energy from both patients and from the relationships with patients, seems essential.

One clinician described this dynamic interchange as an experience of being carried in the healing energy that patients bring with them. Others spoke of a "mutual transfer" of healing energy. So in contrast to the emphasis earlier in this chapter on getting away from one's practice to find sources of renewal, often it is the practice itself and the patient relationships that provide an avenue of self-care. Sometimes clinicians spoke of the privilege of being in the presence of people who could mobilize their own healing resources. This is the phenomenon of recognizing what is healing for each patient and then being willing to be carried along in the stream of the patient's activities. Other practitioners stressed that they began to see at some point in their practices that patients brought with them to the clinic some powerful restorative resources, and that the most important thing was being sure that whatever the medical system offers doesn't get in the way.

A closely related motif in our interviews was the awareness that patients could teach clinicians what worked for them and how this learning can be invigorating and renewing for clinicians. One practitioner put it this way: "I learn things through them that otherwise [I wouldn't know]. I might say to patients: 'I can see this [a particular therapy] isn't working for you.'" Then addressing the interviewer: "I don't have to go out and beat my head against that particular wall. I see it happening right here." Then this practitioner switched to a more positive vein: "Almost everybody who comes in is incredible, but some people are true healers of themselves and don't realize it, and I am kind of drug along in all this. So that to me is a real treat."

Broyard says that in responding to his patients, the doctor can save himself. He concludes: "In learning to talk to his patients, the doctor may talk himself back into loving his work. He has little to lose and everything to gain from letting the sick man into his heart."[8] One of our interviewees spoke with great eloquence about this, noting that the absence of compassion for the patient leads to a downward spiral for the clinician.

> Many clinicians are not trained to understand what is going on inside them. They have a lot of ego involved in the encounter, and the ego is not very compassionate. Clinicians are taught not to bring their heart to work because they fear being swamped by the hurt and suffering of patients. Then they are caught in a cycle. They don't bring their heart, so they can't have compassion for the patient. As a result they are often angry with their patients.

The result of this cycle is that the practitioner's compassion becomes even more remote from patient encounters. By contrast, a primary care practitioner illustrated the rewards of bringing less ego and more heart to work in a story of caring for an elderly patient.

> I have a patient who is 92 and has some health problems, but not many. I say to myself every time I go into the examining room, "Don't give him any medicine. Don't screw it up for him." His wife had dementia and was in a nursing home, and it was a struggle for him. I asked him about it every time because I knew it was on

his mind, even more important than his own health. She died two weeks ago, and he (the patient) said, "What do I do? How am I going to get through this?" I started talking to him, and asked, "What kind of advice are you getting?" He said, "Well, my sons tell me I'll get over it. That I'll get over it in a year. But I don't think so. We've been married 60 years. Every night I had a prayer on my lips for her, for 60 years. I prayed for her every night when I went to bed. So am I going to turn that off after 60 years and forget about her?"

So I said to myself, "Shut up, because you don't have any answers for him." The one primary thing I learned is that I am going to enjoy medicine more if I am a student, and I am still learning from them [patients]. So I said, "I'm not going to be able to tell you how to cope with this, but tell me, what advice do you have for me? I have been married for 30 years. What can I do?" He lit up and leaned forward to grab my hand, that 92-year-old guy. He said, "Call her and tell her you love her. Because I can't do that. I can't tell my wife I love her anymore." And he got teary and I got teary. He grabbed me and said this has been a great visit. I thought, "Wow, this is a bonus. He is going to pay me to come in and give me advice!"

Healing for clinicians can also come from relationships with their patients' families. One intensivist told a story that was deeply moving and defining for him from early in his career. It illustrates the healing impact that a patient's family can have.

When I was a fellow we had a patient we were keeping alive [with lots of invasive technology], and I just loved it. But he had plateaued, not getting any better or any worse. And when I was off for a weekend, the patient died. And I had this real sense of emptiness and failure about what had happened. I had gotten fairly well acquainted with his wife, and she came to the hospital to see me on the Monday after he died—I get tearful every time I think of this—and she told me what the experience was like for her, in making the decision to let him go. She said, "I realized that I was hanging on [to the husband] for me, but I let go for him." And I found that concept to be incredibly helpful in guiding these processes. . . . [I now say to families,] "I'm a physician; I like my patients to get well and go home. That's not what is going to happen, so we need to figure out what to do for him." We [physician and family] have this common sense of failure, that we're not going to get out of this what we want. If we know he's not going to survive—and once we realize we're all in this losing situation together—it makes it much easier to do what we need to do. . . . And that's what I learned from her: often we are hanging on for us, but we have to let go for the patient.

I: That's a powerful lesson.

P: Yeah. I feel forever indebted to that lady who came back in to teach me that lesson.

I: It's interesting that she came back, actually, to see you.

P: Yeah. I'll always wonder if Dr. _____ [chief of service] told her to do that. It was really healing.

The Gift of the Patient

One dimension of the dialectic of healing has to do with the recognition that patients bring with them not only burdens and expectations, suffering and grief, but also gifts for the practitioner. The fundamental gift the patient brings for the clinician is the chance to be a healer. Some of our clinicians talked as if being in the presence of the sick and suffering was a privilege, because it constitutes an exchange of gifts. This dynamic can be understood as a more profound instance of a more usual and mundane exchange of goods and services.

For example, those with broken cars take them to the mechanic, in exchange for money, but also at least for some mechanics, there is the satisfaction of having done a job well, and of having helped someone.

In the common parlance, they have "been of service." Mechanics need the broken car to practice their skills, and the exchange, even if monetary, sometimes rises to something more human and helpful. In similar ways, lawyers need their clients, bankers need their customers, and teachers need their students. But to find the exchange healing or restorative, what the person in need brings in must be seen as a gift that they bear for the person whose help is sought. And of course, instead of cars for repair, the sick bring themselves, the depth of which we recognize by renaming the person as suffering and vulnerable—a "patient." With health practitioners, or at least the best of them, the gift the patient brings is recognized as a possible occasion to be, at least for this one patient, a healer. This exchange of mutual recognition—a reciprocity of needs—has been studied by social scientists for some time. What was emphasized in our interviews is that recognizing the presence of the patient as itself a gift makes it restorative, healing, for the practitioner. One of our interviewees said it definitively:

> The greatest gift you give anybody is your presence, not in the verbal sense [talking], but just being present . . . to sit down on their level and be quiet. That is a gift. It is the greatest gift I can give them. My expertise is not what my gift is. My gift is to be present; and then I help people. But it is a challenge to remember. And it is a beautiful thing, because it is such a privilege. Not many people get to do that. The privilege of being given the gift of another person to you. I get the gift of their lives to me. And you never cease to be amazed by that gift that you get by being there for somebody. They give me the gift of healing, and I give them back my presence. It is amazing how patients really understand that.

It was this recognition of exchange, variously expressed, that made many of our expert clinicians speak about their patients with deep gratitude, and of healthcare practice as a great privilege. They were truly fed by the work itself.

Then there were a few practitioners who were very explicit about how they were fed by seeing the healing exchange with their patients or clients as part of a contribution to a larger mission, making the world "a kinder place."

> Why am I doing this crazy work? . . . Because I can't imagine any greater calling. It's almost like the priesthood for me. It's not a job. It's a calling to give of oneself, of one's heart, fully to another human being . . . in the service of having them be open and be expansive. There is a ripple effect of what I do out of healing presence. Someone else gets that healing, and they become a healing presence, and it becomes a much more loving world. I see it in a really big way. I am but one person. But maybe that starts a wave of compassion and openness for a kinder world, and that is really important to me. . . . I want this world to be a kinder place. I'm going to do what I can to help that along. So I really love what I do. I can't imagine doing anything else.

CONCLUSION: SELF-CARE AND THE CIRCLE OF HEALING

In the opening chapter we delineated eight healing skills practiced by the best clinicians. One of our chief findings was the insistence by our informants that healing does not flow from clinician to patient. It is a feature of the relationship between practitioner and patient, something held between them, or held together or jointly by both parties, as they interact with each other.

In this chapter we have been concerned with delineating what we learned from our informants about how they find health, wholeness, and healing for themselves. Here we have learned that patients themselves sometimes bring their own healing powers into the clinic, and that this can be restorative as well as educational to the practitioner. More often, we were told that the dialectic of interaction that facilitates healing for the patient also brings wholeness and meaning to the practitioner. In short, caring for one's patients is how one cares for oneself. Of course this is a statement with many exceptions and qualifications. But at least some of the time it expresses a basic realization about health care. The opportunity to exercise the defining skills of health care loops back into the practitioner's life, so that as Broyard has said, being a healer for others truly is, in some sense, a way to be whole.

When we began to interview our 50 practitioners we did not expect that practicing the skills we would discover were effective for patient well-being would also be a major part of the clinician's understanding of self-care. But perhaps this is what we should have expected. Healing is not an arrow but a circle. If healing and wholeness are primarily available to us through the quality of relationships, it would have been odd for clinicians to respond to our inquiries about self-care in any other way. This gives new meaning to the instruction "Heal thyself." There is no healing in isolation. The healing of oneself depends, in a fundamental way, on the ability to promote a healing response in others. Or more precisely, the aim is to engage in relationships with patients at a level that can evoke healing powers for both sides of the partnership. Perhaps this can be stated in the imperative mode that was the dominant tone of the skills enumerated in Chapter 1. If you want to take good care of your patients, you must begin by taking good care of yourself.

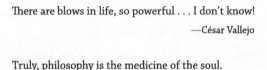

[8]

ETHICS AND MEDICINE: HEALING
THE WOUNDS OF FATE

There are blows in life, so powerful . . . I don't know!

—César Vallejo

Truly, philosophy is the medicine of the soul.

—Cicero

Man's character is his fate.

—Heraclitus

We offer in this concluding chapter one more angle of approach to this matter of healing relationships and the skills of practitioners. We will consider the idea that medicine and ethics are two sets of skills human beings have developed to deal with—to cope with, respond to, recover from—the wounds of fate.

By "wounds of fate" we mean nothing other than those life-changing events and forces outside our control, which are liable to come our way at any moment, on any given day. The unexpected death of a child, a sibling, a spouse, a parent. The loss of a limb, paralysis. Accidents of all kinds, maiming violence, the persistent abuse of a child. Consider also genetic maladies, a vector of fate quite familiar to healthcare practitioners who routinely take medical histories that detail family histories of cancer, of cardiovascular disease, of diabetes. Medical histories that show without speaking it the impact of being born in poverty or into a community built around the dominion of one race over others. There is no one reading these pages who does not know about the blows of fate.

And yet often enough, our practitioners found that these wounds of fate can sometimes result in profound life transformations.

I have one patient who is really amazing. She has vascular disease and I've basically amputated both of her legs—not even any thighs. . . . But she would tell you that she wouldn't even want her legs back now, because of how it's changed her life, how it's made her a different person. . . . If you didn't know this person and you just saw her, you might not know how real a person she is. . . . And about her handicap or her disability . . . the whole language of that. What enables all of us? What disables all of us? How can we call people disabled? Because she's a hell of a lot more enabled than most people I know, and she has no legs. But she is more of what makes a human being than most of us can aspire to.

As another practitioner put it, "I think pain opens your heart."

There are far more occasions, though, where fate simply destroys—at least as far as we can see. And it is in the face of this destruction, and of the lurking possibility of transformation, that we—as individuals, as families, as communities, as nations—learn skills needed to deal with the wounds of life. As far back and as deeply as we can see into our history, two of the fundamental sets of skills human beings have developed to survive the wounds of fate are those of medicine and of ethics. These are not the only skills that serve this purpose, of course. There are those for securing food and shelter; for nurturing children and caring for the dying; for articulating the stories of human life in song and dance, image and word. What we are saying is that medicine and ethics are just as basic and as fundamental as all of these.

To frame this approach to healing relationships, let us step back and review the path we have followed through Chapters 1 through 7. In Chapter 1, we developed a taxonomy of healing skills extrapolated from our interviews with healthcare practitioners. In Chapter 2, we examined ritual patterns that describe the practice of those skills in clinical settings. In Chapter 3, we looked very concretely at how one practitioner developed relationships that were healing. Next, we examined the dynamics of religion and spirituality as they presented themselves in our clinicians' accounts of healing relationships. Then, in Chapter 5, we looked at a variety of patient accounts of how relationships of healing are developed—or aren't—in a variety of healthcare settings and situations. Chapter 6 reviewed some of the evidence from biomedical research that models the power of relationships in the healing process. And in Chapter 7, we listened to our practitioners describe those practices they apply to themselves, for healing in their own lives. Now, we want to bring to the fore questions about healing and the skills of ethics, and about ethics and the process of establishing healing relationships between practitioners and patients.

The question of ethical behavior—of what it is and is not, and how it develops—is unavoidable in discussions of healing relationships. One major facet of ethics concerns the skills involved in establishing, maintaining, and repairing human relationships. Making the case for ethics as a set of life skills to meet and repair the wounds of fate may for some readers mean broadening the usual understanding of ethics as primarily focused on decision processes and their justification. Yet ethics in health care has always involved considering the quality of the relationships between practitioners and their patients.[1]

MASTERING THE SKILLS OF A PRACTITIONER

Our first move in exploring the common territory between medicine and ethics will be to present some basics about skills in general and discuss how they are learned. This will lead into ethics as itself a set of very particular skills. That done, we will be in a position to see more clearly the complementary nature of these two skill sets, medicine and ethics.

What Makes a Skill a Skill?

We have talked about skills throughout this work and have used the word and its grammatical variants in what we take to be their ordinary senses. The following is a list of elements of skillful behavior whose contents are, for the most part, obvious. We are not concerned with a technical definition, nor do we claim the list below is exhaustive, but it gives us enough to explicate and develop our practitioners' comments on what they do as clinicians and how they learned to do what they do.

Skills must be taught
A skill is an ability to do a certain task again and again successfully. Apprentices who come in without skills can be directed to engage in sequences of new behaviors that, if performed properly, will bring about a desired result. Learning skills involves learning (a) new behaviors, (b) the proper sequence of these behaviors, and (c) the ability to recognize what counts as a "desired result." Repetition and trial and error will be central to these learnings. One mark of successful training in a skill is that one can perform it again and again and again, in a wide variety of situations and circumstances.

Skills are socially recognized activities and as such need to be socially validated, named, approved. However "innate" a skill may seem to be, it still requires validation to be counted as a skill. And minimally, this validation is teaching.

Skills entail many more restricted and simpler skills
for their execution
The skill we call "driving a car" comprises an enormous number of component skills. One must be able, for example, to interpret sensory

information rapidly and supplement that with information from the instrument panel; to react quickly in life-or-death situations; to respond physically in a coordinated manner, to the movements of the vehicle; to hold concentration over long periods of time. People who have mastered the skill we call "driving a car" will recognize other subsets of skills involved in "driving a car" that someone without those skills cannot. And the same applies to fighting fires, teaching third-graders, or practicing medicine.

Skills are built hierarchically, progressing from the simple to the complex. Complex skills are dependent on simpler ones. Simple skills make more complex skills available. Practicing simple skills is the best preparation for learning complex skills.

Learning a skill entails developing habits

Habits underlie actual performance of skilled activity. The habit is the skill ingrained into the body, remembered by muscles and cells, and always present and ready to be put into action with a minimum of reflection. Reflection is then typically focused on analyzing the situation in which the skills will be deployed, rather than working through how to perform the various behaviors that constitute the skill.

Skills are taught by recognized authorities—by mentors, teachers, experts—who have demonstrated mastery in teaching the given skill

Attending physicians may be thought of as such masters. And as masters of a particular set of skills to be practiced in specific contexts, they are accepted by apprentices as authorities. Their judgments about what counts as a successful performance of a given skill are at the core of all skills training.

The recognition of an authority is twofold: (1) Masters must be recognized in their field by their colleagues as accomplished performers of the requisite skills, and (2) Masters must be recognized by apprentices as authorities, even if only in a very specific and limited domain (e.g., a particular technique of suturing).

This clinician gives us a description of his own development that includes both of these elements: the recognition of his mentor as a teacher of distinction, and his own recognition of this teacher as his mentor.

    I: Did you have a special mentor?

    P: I did. I came to _____ with no idea that I was going to be a pediatrician, much less an academic pediatrician, much less an academic hematologist and oncologist. But one of the very formative relationships was with _____. I first encountered him between my first and second years. I wanted to stay in town for the summer and was looking for a job. The only thing I could find was a scholarship from the American Cancer Society to do a clinical rotation in the oncology service. So I spent six weeks with _____. He was a pediatric oncologist, and even at the end of that summer I didn't think about being a pediatric oncologist. But I think that even then he had a profound influence on me. I continued to go through medical school and went into pediatrics. I was able to be comfortable with children. And I was able to have difficult conversations with parents and children, because I realized I was helping kids get better. _____ was just a wonderful role model in this regard. A very calm demeanor and very compassionate—just the way he does things. I'm a very different person than he is and my style is quite different. But I think in terms of being a role model, he was clearly the single most influential person, especially in terms of how to interact with patients and families. He's retired, but I still have lunch with him every few weeks. He comes to some of our meetings, and I still have him doing advising.

And then sometimes this mentor, as part of the teaching, will point out and recommend another person with mastery to his students:

I'll say to the students and residents, "What is your reaction to this patient? And why do you think you are reacting that way?" "How do you see Dr. _____ reacting to the patient?" Dr. _____ is able to view each one of these people as human beings with potential, rather than as just a re-admit. And so we try to have a discussion that includes self-awareness, that includes recognizing how you react to patients.

Once again, there is the twofold process. The mentor is recommended by a peer as a teaching authority, and that new mentor is in turn recognized as, and accepted by, the students.

Four Key Elements in Learning and Teaching Skills

1. Observation of skilled performance

From the apprentice's point of view, "observation" means having the skills to be learned demonstrated and named. "This is 'x', and this is not." The skill must be displayed clearly and named clearly, not just displayed rapidly and assuredly. So the greatest practitioners are often not the greatest teachers. The other essential aspect of observation for the student is learning how to recognize a proper outcome, how to know one has succeeded. How does one know one has taken a proper patient history, or that one has found what can be known from palpating a liver or listening to a heart?

> I think a lot of the basic skills you learn by watching role models, both good and bad. In the very beginning, there's people that you see that really seem to do a good job of this. Sometimes, as a student and as a resident, it's difficult to know exactly how or why they're doing it, but you can at least see that it's effective. And that motivates you to try to reach that same level. You also see super-clear role models of things that you will not do, and that sticks with you, too.

From the mentor's point of view, being observed by students entails the very particular skill of recognizing, in the flow of events in a given day, "teachable moments." The best of these moments are the opportunities to model behaviors in situations that arise unexpectedly.

> Sometimes when I see that a patient is angry with me, and I have students in the room, I am thinking in the back of my mind: "This is great." This is a teachable moment for these students. I don't know if I am going to deal with this the right way, but at least the students can see how I deal with it. Then they can reflect on it and see if I have done well or I haven't. Usually you know if you've done well. If you walk into an angry patient and they leave a more satisfied patient. They still might be disgruntled, but maybe they are less disgruntled than they were before.

These are also moments that entail a certain amount of risk for the mentor: "I don't know if I am going to deal with this the right way." But that risking, in and of itself, teaches students an essential lesson about the vulnerability of being a clinician.

2. Performances of skills overseen and reviewed by mentors

Observation of a skill is one thing; the correct performance of it is another. The gap between observation and mastery is filled by efforts to perform the observed skill and critique of those efforts and their outcomes by a master of the skills. This detailed example offered by one clinician gives us a very clear picture of this dynamic.

> A colleague was doing a course for people who were interested in teaching communication in the institution. There were about six physicians going through this. And he pointed out to me, in a fairly difficult role-playing exercise, that I had a tendency to respond to a patient's complaint with some plan of how to fix it, rather than just stopping for a minute and allowing the patient to express the emotions.

There is the performance of the skill in front of a mentor that this clinician has accepted as an authority. This acceptance entails, as a precondition for this type of learning, setting aside control and protection. Then comes the critique of the performance.

> The role playing involved another physician enacting their most difficult patient. So I had to try to communicate with this old person who had chronic pain and kept coming in for visits. When this "patient" would talk about the pain, the default was to say, "We're going to work on this; we're going to adjust your medications."

And after the critique came the suggestion of new behaviors that will improve subsequent performance of the skill.

> And he [the mentor] taught me to step back for a second and say, "Tell me a little bit about the pain. How is it affecting your daily routine?" Those kinds of things. Not just always jumping to try to fix it, but just doing what a normal person who can't fix it would say: "Boy, that sounds really tough. Tell me, how is it working out?" Doing what a nonphysician would who doesn't have the end goal of saying, "I can make it go away."

In this case, the suggestion was to break out of the professional role as clinician, and the specific assumptions and skills that that role is governed by, and go back into the "ordinary" world of human interactions and relationships. The ensuing task for the clinician is incorporating the new behaviors into his daily practice of medicine.

> And so I started to do that a little bit more with certain emotions or complaints of pain or things like that—just taking a second to reflect back to the patient that that sounds difficult, before jumping to some kind of game plan to make it go away. That's a very specific thing that he brought out for me a few years ago.

What follows is another round of observations, this time by the clinician. And there remains the possibility of returning to the mentor for further critique and further instruction—*for the process of learning a skill never ends.* There are always nuances of behavior or context to master, always supplementary and complementary skills to acquire.

3. Trial and error
After new behaviors have been rehearsed comes the process of building them into new habits that improve the daily performance.

> Unless a doctor can recognize certain symptoms, e.g., the accentuation of the second sound of the pulmonary artery, there is no use in his reading the description of syndromes of which this symptom forms a part. He must personally know that symptom, and he can learn this only by repeatedly being given cases for auscultation in which the symptom is authoritatively known to be present, side by side with other cases in which it is authoritatively known to be absent, until he has fully realized the difference between them and can demonstrate his knowledge practically to the satisfaction of an expert.[2]

Repetition runs alongside trial and error:

> I: How did you learn this way of managing? Did you have clinical mentors, or was it more trial and error?
> P: A lot of it's trial and error. But I think the big thing is that you try to figure out what you can do to do the best job possible. Again, it's very important for me that the process is the right one.

"The right one." This is what is learned from the mentor; this is the goal of habits that support the execution of the skill.

4. The use of imperatives
"Do this." "Don't do it that way." "Try it this way instead." "Yes, that's it. Do it again." Skills *can only be learned* by following and trusting a recognized master's imperatives.

That's one thing that I'm trying to teach my brother, who's joining my practice as a new clinician. When he first started, I had him adjust me. And his hands were shaking a little, and a little unsure. I said, "Wow, let's talk about that. When you put your hands on somebody, take like a few really slow deep breaths. Really try and control that shaking, okay? Because you don't want that."

Only recognized authorities can validate the learning of the apprentice. "Yes, this person now has the skill." And as we will see later, in medicine it is often the patient who is this "authority."

Skills Are Practiced in Specific Contexts—and Have to Be Learned There

Mastery of a skill involves recognizing the appropriate context for practicing a given skill—the right time and place and in the presence of the right people. For example, placing a needle is a very different thing for giving an injection, establishing an IV, completing a liver biopsy, doing an acupuncture treatment. All are skilled behaviors, but enormously different skills when exercised in their particular context. Likewise, the exercise of skill with needles will be very different when speaking of doing a carpet repair, stitching a canvas seam, learning to knit, or doing needlepoint. Yet in every case one might speak of skills with needles.

And then there is what we may call the "geographical" context, which is always very specific. Where is a skill to be learned? And where is it to be practiced?

You wonder how many of these little things students and residents pick up on. I think they're very important. And so the first couple of encounters with a patient I see with a student, I do try to let them know. Sometimes in front of the patient and student and resident, I will articulate some of these things. I'll tell the student, "It is always a good idea to wash your hands in front of the patient." And I've got my patient right here. The patient sometimes will say: "Yeah, that is really important." They were teaching the students: "Always do that." Or sometimes: "Don't make your patient wait like your Dr. _____ does."

The specificity of context for the exercise of a skill is an aspect of its performance that will be of considerable importance later when we turn to examine further skills that bind ethics and medicine together.

FINDING THE MENTOR

We turn now to the question of who teaches the healthcare practitioner about healing relationships. Some of these masters will be obvious and others not. And, correspondingly, some of these relational skills we expect from practitioners come readily to mind, while others are more subtle. Yet these mostly unnoticed skills may turn out to be among the most important ones when it comes to practitioners establishing healing relationships with their patients.

Medical Education—Positive and Negative Models

We would expect, we should certainly hope, that clinicians will have found significant models for establishing healing relationships with their patients during their professional training.

The supervisors that I had that I respected were the ones who had a very human approach to taking care of patients. They listen to them. They go the extra mile.

What that "extra mile" is will vary from situation to situation, from context to context.

We had a patient at the VA who was dying of cancer and there wasn't anything to do for him. Just check and make sure the nurses are giving him his pain meds and, "Is there anything you need?" When you're doing rounds, you've already got ten times more patients to see than you have time for. Stop by, poke your head in, "Hey, Mr. Smith." Or you might not. You might just bypass the room altogether. But we had this one guy who would make us stop. We'd all have to sit down in the room to show Mr. Smith that we weren't in a rush. And this guy said to us, "You know, the only thing we have to give that patient is time. The only thing we can do for him is to give him some of our time." And that always stuck with me. That's the kind of stuff you can model.

Many of our interviewees were fortunate enough to find exemplary mentors to observe and to emulate. But unfortunately, many interviewees found that often in their medical education the most significant teaching about how to relate to patients was done by what one called "reverse mentors":

In terms of mentors, no, I didn't have anyone alongside me that I looked at and said, "I want to be like him." What I found was people in a reverse mentor role: "I don't want to be that way."

As students they were looking for models. But, again:

But there were very few role models that I would ever want to emulate. . . although they were technically skilled and knew things and were great researchers. . . none of them, very few, were models as human beings that I could really look up to. Very few.

Family

For many of our practitioners, it was family members who were their most significant mentors when it came to establishing relationships with their patients.

My family is very important—we were just raised to be very respectful and try to see the other person's point of view, even if you don't agree with it. We were kind of just raised that way.

There is direct carryover into clinical practice.

> I: What does the patient feel when the physician comes out to greet them and shakes their hand and walks together with them. . . .
>
> P: Yeah, I always invite the patient into the office. But what you're hearing from me now are things my mother taught me. Let's be truthful.
>
> I: Right. Not things you learned during your residency.

The foundations for relationships with patients, indeed with all other people, were laid early for many of our extraordinary practitioners.

Patients

Far and away the most important mentors for clinicians, especially in terms of our study, are their patients. This enormous and heterogeneous group of people have many, many different types of lessons and skills to teach practitioners. Sometimes they have to do with the "meaning of medicine", sometimes with simply "being human", and sometimes, more grandly, with the "meaning of life."

> People are amazing, individuals are amazing. And I think that is the inherent joy of medicine. We have an opportunity to be wise beyond our capacity, because people tell us everything. They tell us their mistakes and they tell us about their joy. They instruct us.

And sometimes the "meaning of death":

> I've learned a lot from patients in the way they approach death, and I have much less fear about it for myself.

There is, then, instruction in what may be called "life skills." And there is also instruction that has specific impact on clinical practice.

We have used the following story once before, in our discussion of the dialectic of healing in Chapter 7. But it provides such a wonderful example of a physician learning from a member of a patient's family that we are going to pick up one piece of it again.

> And then she [the wife of the man who died] said to me, "I realized that I was hanging on for me, but I let go for him." And I found that concept to be incredibly helpful in guiding these processes . . .when I have a family and they know that I'm coming in there to say that it's time to pull the plug. . . . So I say: "We're not going to get out of this what we want . . . so now, if he were sitting at this table, what would he be telling us?" And that's what I learned from her: often we're hanging on for us, but we let go for the patient.

Repeatedly, our practitioners said they learned such lessons from their patients. Their medical education may not have given them much direct training in healing relationships, but their patients did—and still do.

Yet there remains a far more fundamental reason that patients are essential mentors for clinicians, one that reaches into the heart of both medicine and ethics. And it is this: only patients can teach the practitioner about vulnerability and about what it is like to partner with, and take some portion of responsibility for, a vulnerable life, a wounded life. No professional mentors can do this, by definition, in their role as practitioners, teachers, and authorities in the practice of medicine. In these matters, the masters are the people who have suffered, who have been wounded.

> One of the most difficult things I've dealt with recently is a patient who's a long-standing acquaintance. He's my go-to plumber, and he's also been my patient. No problems over

the years. He called to say he was having some chest discomfort and needed to be seen. He doesn't call very often, so we worked him in; it was late on a Thursday afternoon, and I looked at his X-ray. It was horrible. He had this new lung mass. Huge. Big as a grapefruit, and his previous X-ray had been normal. That was particularly difficult for me.

By simply standing before the practitioner as people who have suffered, who have been wounded, patients *are* the mentors. They are the great teachers of woundedness to physicians.

I had this one boy who was the same age as my son with an 80 percent body burn, who amazingly survived. But you know it just broke my heart. And so I stopped at the market on the way in to buy candy.

By his sheer presence the patient is saying, "This is what a wounded life is, what it looks like. Are you looking? Can you look? Will you look? And if you look, will you see?"

If I sense early in the conversation that for instance a breast cancer patient who has had an outside biopsy and knows that they have the diagnosis of cancer . . . so they're coming in with that information. If you see, right up front, that they are very scared and tense, just talking about that, just very openly saying, "You look very scared; I would imagine that this would be very frightening for you to know this."

And to the degree that the clinician continues to stand there, and continues to fully see and hear, to that degree he shares those wounds.

So last week there was a 31-year-old patient who fell from an elevator shaft. He almost died but not quite, and he wasn't going to regain consciousness. His heart was beating, he's on a vent, and I wanted to come out with the DNR. And the family didn't want to hear it, and I knew they didn't. . . . But it needed to be done and . . . on that case I pushed, and I pushed really hard. And I did it not because I wanted to be right or wrong, but because I felt that it wasn't in the patient's best interest to be resuscitated. There was nothing to resuscitate back.

And sharing the wounds creates a bond, a mutual recognition at a human level of what one of the practitioners called "Just a pure human predicament."

One of the things I consciously do is I try to listen hard, and I try to convey to the patient that even on saying hello, as far as I'm concerned, from my point of view, "We're in this together." Just a pure human predicament.

We are both human beings. We are both vulnerable. I am here now with you, sharing that fundamental aspect of being human—which is the inevitability of vulnerability.

When the patient is a member of the practitioner's family, a whole new arena for being instructed about vulnerability opens up. This shift, as many clinicians have described, brings huge and immediate changes. As this intensivist relates,

P: Eventually, they roll my dad into the ICU and they get him hooked up and we walk into the room. Everything in the room was familiar: every piece of equipment, all the monitors, the flashing lights, which . . . that was where I live. But this was my dad, and it was this sense of, "What is going on here?" It was really a strange experience for me. . . .

I: I can imagine.

P: Because everything was so familiar, every piece of it, except who it's hooked to. And then I found myself, "But what does all this stuff mean, about this guy?" Which is what the patients—the families do. They come in and see all this stuff, and the only thing they recognize is their loved one. They're wondering, "But what does all this stuff around here mean?"

The demands made on patients and families can be seen in an entirely different light when the practitioner herself becomes the patient:

I had a rollover Jeep accident when I was a resident. I went to the local ER, and was sent home. I came to work the next day and asked for the CT scan. I ended up getting an operation on my abdomen, because I had a torn loop of intestine from the impact and multiple rib fractures. . . . So nothing actually that had any kind of long-term consequence, but it did make me appreciate a little bit, in that immediate recovery period, of what it was like to lose the integrity of your body.

One has been shifted from one social and existential class to another. One has become a member of the class of the wounded. And by virtue of this shift, the practitioner is able to recognize in new ways what it means to inhabit and to display the vulnerability of all bodies, of all lives.

Where have our practitioners found their mentors? In families and communities; in medical school; among patients, including those times they or a close family member were patients. And why is it so important to find mentors? Because this is the way skills are learned, the only way skills are learned. This is the case whether those practitioner skills are what we think of as "technical," suturing or the placement of needles in acupuncture, or "relational," how to deal with angry families or patients who have just experienced major trauma.

We indicated at the beginning of this chapter that we intended to approach ethics as a set of skills, as we have approached the process of establishing healing relationships in health care. It is time now to turn to that territory and examine ethics and philosophy in light of what we have said about skills and mentoring.

ETHICS AS THE PRACTICE OF LIFE

Long before the modern notion of philosophical ethics as problem-solving became dominant, ethics meant the art of living one's life in a certain way.

> The philosophical act is not situated merely on the cognitive level, but on that of the self and of being. It is a progress which causes us to *be* more fully, and makes us better. It is a conversion which turns our entire life upside down, changing the life of the person who goes through it.[3]

This is taken from Pierre Hadot's classic work, *Philosophy as a Way of Life*. And how is this radical "conversion" to be brought about?

> Spiritual exercises can best be observed in the context of Hellenistic and Roman schools of philosophy. The Stoics, for instance, declared explicitly that philosophy, for them, was an "exercise." In their view, philosophy did not consist in teaching an abstract theory—much less in the exegesis of texts—but rather in the art of living.[4]

Coming fresh off our examination of skills, we have immediate questions here. What is this *exercise* of philosophy, where and how is it taught, and who does the teaching? And, finally, what does it mean to think of the exercise of philosophy as, fundamentally, a way of living? There is also the larger frame of this chapter to keep in mind. What can this ancient practice of philosophy teach us about responding to the wounds of fate? And what about that practice parallels, and complements, medicine as a response to those same "blows"?

Let us continue with Hadot and ask how a philosophical life would manifest itself concretely. A life shaped by this exercise would show, Hadot says,

> ...in the order of inner discourse and of spiritual activity: meditation, dialogue with oneself, examination of conscience,

exercises of the imagination . . . or in the order of action and of daily behavior, like the mastery of oneself, indifference toward indifferent things, the fulfillment of the duties of social life in Stoicism, the discipline of desires in Epicureanism.[5]

Most all of this is lost in the 21st-century definitions of both philosophy and ethics. Philosophers are now almost completely identified as academics, university professors who are rewarded for theorizing and are generally not known for speaking to a broad public audience. This accounts, in part, for the initial puzzlement when philosophy as a response to the wounds of fate is proposed.[6]

The ancient teaching is that philosophy and ethics are about the way one chooses to live as a whole, on a quotidian basis, and the exercises, tasks, and teachings that will enable that life to be considered good, authentic, and worthwhile. Take, for example, the most basic teaching of Epictetus, that one must draw a sharp distinction between the things that are within one's powers and the many things that are not. And that our well-being finally rests on not attaching oneself inordinately to things one does not control. This is usually combined in Stoic philosophy with gratitude for life and a deep sense of civic responsibility. Or, to take an example from the best known of the ancient philosophers, a Socratic dialogue is a spiritual exercise practiced with the purpose of giving appropriate attention to oneself, knowing and taking care of those aspects of self that are most important. Ethical dialogue, as it is put on display by Plato, is precisely an exercise in authentic presence of the self to itself, and to the self of others. These dialogues are not meant to problem-solve, but to form character. Their goal is to arrive at the truths of how to live— how to flourish by attending to one's soul.

Hadot's presentation of the process of philosophical formation includes three major components of interest to us: (1) the exercises used to teach students the philosophical way of living, (2) the schools where training took place, and (3) the goals of that training, of those schools. The reader will note where his account of this formation intersects our taxonomy of skills. It is also to be noted that the effort to explicate ancient philosophy as a way of life involves expanding the vocabulary customarily used to depict philosophy, and training in philosophy. This sometimes awkward effort is itself an essential step in approaching philosophy primarily as a matter of skills, and not of analysis, theories, and problem-solving.[7]

How, then, are these philosophers trained? What skills must they master? What exercises must be undertaken? The answers to these questions will vary depending on which teaching tradition one is referring to. We will take our illustrative examples from exercises central for Stoic schools.[8]

For the Stoics, attentiveness and the disciplining of mental states is the core of formation. One crucial skill is the mastery of mind by incorporating into one's life certain "fundamental principles."

> The preparatory exercise (*melete*) allows us to be ready at the moment when an unexpected—and perhaps dramatic—circumstance occurs. In the exercise called *praemeditatio malorum* [premeditation of misfortunes] we are to represent to ourselves poverty, suffering, and death. We must confront life's difficulties face to face, remembering that they are not evils, since they do not depend on us.[9]

Exercises are done to prepare the philosopher for the "dramatic circumstances," for what we referred to at the beginning of this chapter as the wounds of fate. And there are specific exercises designed to prepare one for specific wounds—that of death in the example above. Another regular preparatory exercise included what in our time might be thought of as a pragmatics reading. We are to approach texts in such a way as to "engrave striking maxims in our memory." Such thoroughly appropriated maxims will then be ready for use in meeting those severe challenges "which are, after all, part of the course of nature."[10] We "learn by heart," we engrave into the core of the body, certain teachings so that no matter what happens to us, we can respond to events out of those teachings, and not out of immediate self-centeredness driven by the passions. Certain genres of discourse were found to be especially effective in putting forward the needed "maxims."

What we need are persuasive formulae or arguments (*epilogismoi*), which we can repeat to ourselves in difficult circumstances, so as to check movements of fear, anger, or sadness.[11]

And then there are the Stoics' social exercises emphasizing self-mastery in all one's dealings with others and in the performance of one's social duties. In this training, "one very simple principle is always recommended: begin practicing on easier things, so as gradually to acquire stable, solid habit." This development of habits, as we noted earlier in this chapter, is a hallmark of training in skills. Habits shape our immediate responses, responses that occur "before we have time to think." Which means, in the context of ethics and ethical development, "before we would have a chance to engage in ethical discussion or reflection that might guide a reaction or shape a judgment." And yet it is just in such immediate responses that the bulk of ethical behavior is found.[12]

The specific location, institution, or context for the teaching of these skills was the philosophical schools. But, again, we must work hard to get past the notions of training in philosophy sponsored by modern philosophy and reach into territory more commonly approached these days as "spiritual disciplines," as that type of "meditation" several of our practitioners have spoken of in previous chapters. "In all philosophical schools, the goal pursued in these exercises is self-realization and improvement." And why pursue such a goal? The matter may be couched in modern philosophical terminology as "existential": "All schools agree that man, before his philosophical conversion, is in a state of unhappy disquiet." And why so unhappy? "Consumed by worries, torn by passions, he does not live a genuine life, nor is he truly himself." In this state one is distracted from oneself and what one could be, degraded by and in one's own life. And the promise is equally radical: "All schools also agree that man can be delivered from this state."[13]

Here Hadot is of course referring to literal "schools"—places where students go to learn by performing specific exercises given to them by recognized mentors. In these schools apprentices undertook a process of self-transformation under the guidance of a master.

And the master's writings were developed in these schools and aimed at the formation of his students, not the development of abstract arguments or systems. Teaching was focused on particulars and dealt with specific examples and specific students. Again, these are hallmarks of the teaching skills elucidated above.[14] And the goal of these exercises, the purpose of these schools?

> Each school had its own therapeutic method, but all of them linked their therapeutics to a profound transformation of the individual's mode of seeing and being. The object of spiritual exercises is precisely to bring about this transformation.[15]

And what imagery is used to depict this transformation, these therapeutics?

> "We must concern ourselves with the healing of our own lives." Epicurus
> "Truly, philosophy is the medicine of the soul." Cicero
> "Vain is the word of that philosopher which does not heal any suffering." Epicurus
> "The philosopher's school is a clinic." Epictetus[16]

Philosophy as medicine, its teachers as practitioners, its schools as clinics, its goal as healing.

With this in hand, we are ready now to turn back to look at ethics and at medicine as sets of skills, there to be mastered, that can help us respond to human vulnerability, to human woundedness. A wounding so universal as to be an incontrovertible strand of human fate.

HEALING SKILLS AS CHARACTER TRAITS

We have provided this excursus into ancient traditions of ethics precisely because it is not just ancient, but completely contemporary—alive and well in the minds of the practitioners we interviewed.

Ethics, to our practitioners, is decidedly not theory and is only partly problem-solving. Ethics has primarily to do with how to live one's professional and personal life, in the context of daily relationships. It is about helping to heal the wounds they encounter, in both themselves and their patients. After hearing the descriptions of healing and relational skills our practitioners offered, we frequently asked them what they thought the exercise of these skills had to do with ethics. On one occasion our query about the ethical import of these skills met with a blank incredulity. The passage below will stand in for many others in which the practitioner saw no difference between the skills of healing and the practice of ethics. Here the interviewee is reading a copy of the questions we had given him in advance:

P: "Would you describe any aspect of your relationship to your patients as ethical?" Is that a typo? Do I describe the relationships as ethical?

I: Obviously you do. The thing that . . .

P: I am confused. You don't mean unethical. I would have to think about if there are any unethical things I do. I like to think everything I do is ethical. It's hopefully all ethical. I squirm if I start to wonder if there is something unethical. Do I need to talk about that?

I: No, no. You've done great—that's a great answer.

To our practitioners, everything they had been describing to us was ethics. As Pellegrino points out it in the epigram that opens Chapter 1, "At the center of medical ethics is the healing relationship."

We return now to Table 1.2 (Chapter One above, pp. 23-4). This table, as you recall, depicted a sequence of eight skills described by our extraordinary practitioners—indeed enjoined by them—as ones essential for the development of healing relationships. What we want to tease out in this section is the idea that each of these skills may be thought of as associated with a character trait—and that these character traits are themselves skills.

Our practitioners say that every aspect of their practice involves ethics, no matter how "value-neutral," purely technical, scientific, or "evidence-based" it may appear to be. And given the minimal assumption that ethics has fundamentally to do with human relationships, we would expect to find that the eight sets of skills essential for building healing relationships would be themselves ethical in nature. Let us then propose that each of the eight skill sets can be elucidated by associating it with certain character traits.[17] Some of our choices of traits will be more obvious than others. But we think the pairings below capture the spirit of the many ways our practitioners spoke about relationships that heal. Our eight items range from very simple changeable and easily measurable behaviors (eye contact, posture, listening without interrupting, speaking with less jargon) to huge lifetime projects (being brave, taking risks, being loyal). One advantage of associating each set of skills in developing healing relationships with a character trait is that such an association emphasizes the life-long nature of the learning these skills entail and demand.[18]

Take courage as an example. This is a trait whose association with its corresponding skill set may look less obvious than some of the others on the list. The crux is that the practitioner's willingness to walk into the suffering of his or her patients again and again is itself courage. Opening oneself to suffering, standing with a person who is wounded, always involves risks—physical, mental, emotional, spiritual. Taking such a risk on occasion involves sporadic acts of courage. Taking them continually, as a part of one's daily practice, one's daily life—this is to have courage, to have courage as a habit, to have courage as a trait of one's character.

Let us, as another example, follow this detailed account given by a neonatologist of humility as a skill set that can be taught and can be learned.

> P: Another thing I think is important is humility. I'm not too good to open a door or roll a patient back into a room. I'm not too proud to wipe the snot off a crying mother. I'm not too

Table 8.1

Healing Skills	Character Traits
1. Do the little things	**Humility**
• Introduce yourself and everyone on the team	
• Greet everybody in the room	
• Shake hands; smile; sit down; make eye contact	
• Give your undivided attention	
• Be human, be personable	
2. Take time	**Patience**
• Be still	
• Be quiet	
• Be interested	
• Be present	
3. Be open and listen	**Courage**
• Be vulnerable	
• Be brave	
• Face the pain	
• Look for the unspoken	
4. Find something to like, to love	**Compassion**
• Take the risk	
• Stretch yourself and your world	
• Think of your family	
5. Remove barriers	**Justice**
• Practice humility	
• Pay attention to power and its differentials	
• Create bridges	
• Be safe and make welcoming spaces	

(Continued)

Table 8.1 CONTINUED

Healing Skills	Character Traits
6. Let the patient explain	**Empathy**
• Listen for what and how patients understand	
• Listen for the fear and for the anger	
• Listen for expectations and for hopes	
7. Share authority	**Respect**
• Offer guidance	
• Get permission to take the lead	
• Support patients' efforts to heal themselves	
• Be confident	
8. Be committed and trustworthy	**Integrity**
• Do not abandon	
• Invest in trust	
• Be faithful	
• Be thankful	

good to do any of those things that the lowest-ranked employee of the hospital does. If I see a need, I'll do what it takes to meet it. I don't mind getting dirty and getting down.... There's no shame in dirty work.

I: But this must send a powerful message that, as a team, everybody who's involved in the care has a kind of fundamental human equality.

P: I think it does. If a leader moves in that direction, everybody else is more likely to.

That is a description of the kinds of things that a person who has mastered the core skills of humility does. It includes being willing to "do the little things"—in this case things often thought beneath the role or dignity of the practitioner. Notice now who are named as mentors.

> I: Did you have important teachers for these things that are important to you? Or were they things that you learned through trial and error?
>
> P: It's not all learned. I came with some of it, and I learned some it from others. Being a farm person is huge. And coming from a small community. All I knew were humble farm people. And humility is just totally ingrained in that type of people. Humility comes before anything; in fact, probably too much so.

She identifies the community where she was raised as, collectively, her fundamental teacher of humility. Her first models were found there.

> And then, I have watched people, but not necessarily physician peers. That is not where I learned that from. I can't even give you an example of a physician peer who taught me about being on an equal level with the patient. And humility: I've learned that from housekeepers. And probably the greatest teacher is the respiratory therapist I work with, a man that I've worked with for 21 years. He is the most quiet, unobtrusive, humble person I've ever known, and thus the most powerful man I've ever met. He has no clue he's that powerful, but his behaviors ripple through every layer. Humility is probably the single greatest character trait.

We learned above, in our general discussion of skills, that it is always critical to find out who the mentors are, who the masters are, if we are to truly grasp the nature of the skill at hand. This is also true when it comes to those skills that, when mastered, show that a person has a given character trait. For this clinician, the mentors here have not been physicians. The masters of humility for her have been housekeepers and a respiratory therapist.

We are well aware that by "the norms of argument," nothing is "established" by making a list that associates healing skills with character traits. But guided by Hadot, we are not looking here for proofs, but for further practical guidance. Tables and lists of traits like ours are at once rhetorical devices, pedagogical strategies and mnemonic methods for formation and edification, and have been used in teaching traditions the world over for millennia.

These associations of skills and traits also have the advantage of inviting further exploration. In particular, we would emphasize the potential importance of the idea that ethics may be best approached as a matter of learning and practicing sets of skills, and the idea that the character traits can be useful ways for naming such skill sets. Also, and to our purpose in this book, there is the possibility that these ideas may provide guidance for those seeking to develop effective means and methods for training future clinicians in the skills and habits necessary for establishing, on a regular basis, healing relationships.

Let us review: We came into this chapter on medicine and ethics after thorough consideration of what 50 extraordinary practitioners had to say about healing, relationships, and the meaning of medicine—and by way of that, about their understandings of the balance and value of life itself. Moving through the chapter, with assistance from our clinicians, and from Pierre Hadot's account of ancient philosophy, we have urged that ethics be understood as itself a discipline and art of healing in a way that parallels, as well as infuses, medicine. We have claimed that when this is recognized, the deeper recognition may follow that medicine and ethics are two complementary sets of skills that enable human beings to respond to the inevitable wounds of fate.

The terms "fate" and "wounds" may seem overwrought for the daily round of medicine, and of our lives. It is true that the wounds we tend to speak of, the matters of fate we tend to recall, are the more egregious disruptions of the order of a patient's world. This chapter opened with just such examples. But it is no contradiction to turn and point out that it is in the smallness that run the most fundamental lines of one's life. And it is just these lines that have commonly been called fate. Further, it is the case that certain wounds unfold only in small steps. Some of these are called "chronic conditions." Others include the slow course of some cancers, and incremental damage to liver or kidneys. At a certain point, though, even without the dramatic blows that come to all, the sequence of small imbalances and rebalancings reveals the course of a person's life.

Turn this another way: Illness is not optional—though some people are more obviously affected than others. Neither is medicine optional—though for some people a formalized healthcare system may not be necessary. Illness is not exceptional; it is natural and normal. And so medicine is not the exception, but the rule. Healing is likewise part of this cycle—natural, normal, and inevitable. The body is subject, as all living things are, to imbalance and wounding. But it also has that fundamentally mysterious capacity, as all living things do, and as noted by so many of our clinicians, to restore balance and to heal. Consider a life, then, as a series of healings.

If Cicero could speak of philosophical schools as clinics, then we may perhaps speak of clinics as philosophical schools. Clinics are places to learn ways of living a new life. Most often these will be "little learnings": "Do this and your cough will go away." "If I do this, your arm will mend." But so often the teachings get more complex: "Let us help you lose that weight. We can help you change your eating habits. We can help you address the emotional wounds underlying those habits." And then there is the time for dying, and for all the learning that process can provide. Quite a number of our clinicians described their care for their patients in terms of these very kinds of teaching.

In such schools, such clinics, practitioners and their patients teach each other about medicine and healing—and thus, necessarily, about ethics and character as ways of living. Somewhat hidden is the fact that clinicians also teach their patients about relational skills, or fail to. Also mostly hidden is the fact that clinicians can, if they will, learn relational skills from their patients. To be sure, as with all schools, some teachers are good and nurturing, and others are quite a bit less so. And like schools, some facilities are better designed and equipped than others. But the core teaching of the clinic about human fate is everywhere the same: Illness is inevitable. Healing is universal. The rhythm of the two, distinctive for each one of us, is one of the fundamentals of our lives. And moving gracefully with that rhythm is a matter of medicine, and of ethics.

NOTES

Chapter 1

The epigraphs to this chapter come from Rachel Remen, quoted in Krista Tippett, *Speaking of Faith* (New York: Penguin Books, 2008), p. 213, and Edmund D. Pellegrino, *Humanism and the Physician* (Knoxville: University of Tennessee Press, 1979), p. 123.

1. Howard Brody, *Placebos and the Philosophy of Medicine: Clinical, Conceptual, and Ethical Issues* (Chicago: University of Chicago Press, 1980).
2. Daniel E. Moerman, *Meaning, Medicine, and the "Placebo Effect"* (New York: Cambridge University Press, 2002).
3. Pellegrino, *Humanism and the Physician*, pp. 117–29.
4. A rare and very interesting exception to this dearth of studies is the one led by John Scott. See John G. Scott, Deborah Cohen, Barbara DiCicco-Bloom, William L. Miller, Kurt C. Stange, and Benjamin F. Crabtree, "Understanding Healing Relationships in Primary Care," *Annals of Family Medicine* 6 (2008): 315–22.
5. See, for example, John L. Coulehan and Marian R. Block, *The Medical Interview: Mastering Skills for Clinical Practice*, 4th ed. (Philadelphia: F. A. Davis, 2001); J. Andrew Billings and John D. Stoeckle, *The Clinical Encounter: A Guide to the Medical Interview and Case Presentation*, 2nd ed. (St. Louis: Mosby, 1999); and Elliot G. Mishler, *The Discourse of Medicine: Dialectics of Medical Interviews* (Norwood, NJ: Ablex, 1984).
6. Eric J. Cassell, *Talking with Patients*, vol. 1: *The Theory of Doctor-Patient Communication* (Cambridge, MA: MIT Press, 1985).
7. Malcolm Gladwell, *Blink: The Power of Thinking Without Thinking* (New York: Little, Brown, 2005).

8. Frederic W. Platt, David L. Gaspar, John L. Coulehan, Lucy Fox, Andrew J. Adler, W. Wayne Weston, Robert C. Smith, and Moira Stewart, "'Tell Me about Yourself': The Patient-Centered Interview," *Annals of Internal Medicine* 134 (2001): 1079–85.

9. Pellegrino, *Humanism and the Physician*, p. 123.

10. Howard B. Beckman and Richard M. Frankel, "The Effect of Physician Behavior on the Collection of Data," *Annals of Internal Medicine* 101 (1984): 692–96.

11. See here the work of Rita Charon and Martha Montello—for example, Rita Charon, *Narrative Medicine: Honoring the Stories of Illness* (New York: Oxford University Press, 2006), and Rita Charon and Martha Montello, eds., *Stories Matter: The Role of Narrative in Medical Ethics* (New York: Routledge, 2002).

12. Reynolds Price, *A Whole New Life: An Illness and a Healing* (New York: Atheneum, 1994).

13. Jerome Bruner, "Narratives of Human Plight: A Conversation with Jerome Bruner," in Charon and Montello, *Stories Matter*, p. 4.

14. Jerome Groopman, *How Doctors Think* (Boston: Houghton Mifflin, 2007).

Chapter 2

1. Our understanding of this pattern draws, as does that of so many others, on the work of Arnold van Gennep and Victor Turner. The classics are Arnold van Gennep, *The Rites of Passage*, trans. Monika B. Vizedom and Gabrielle L. Caffee (Chicago: University of Chicago Press, 1960), and Victor Turner, *The Ritual Process: Structure and Anti-Structure* (Hawthorne, NY: Aldine, 1969).

 See also the work of Robert L. Moore on ritual and rites of passage. We especially appreciate his emphasis on the importance of the boundary around the container and on the role of a designated leader in establishing and holding the container. See Robert L. Moore, "Ritual, Sacred Space, and Healing: The Psychoanalyst as Ritual Elder," in *Liminality and Transitional Phenomena*, ed. Nathan Schwartz-Salant and Murray Stein (Wilmette, IL: Chiron, 1991), pp. 13–32, and Robert L. Moore, "Contemporary Psychotherapy as Ritual Process: An Initial Reconnaissance," *Zygon* 18, no. 3 (1983): 283–94.

2. We will use the terms "rite" and "ritual" interchangeably and in what we understand to be in keeping with common usage: a recurrent, patterned set of social behaviors that mark and facilitate key passages in human life (e.g., childbirth, puberty, marriage, death). See also Chapter 4.

3. Arthur Kleinman's work is essential for approaching this territory. See especially his *Patients and Healers in the Context of Culture: An Exploration of the Borderland between Anthropology, Medicine, and Psychiatry* (Berkeley: University of California Press, 1980).

    Among many, many studies on rites and medicine, see the particularly valuable research of Sjaak van der Geest, such as Sjaak van der Geest, "Sacraments in the Hospital: Exploring the Magic and Religion of Recovery," *Anthropology and Medicine* 12, no. 2 (2005): 135–50, and Sjaak van der Geest and Kaja Finkler, "Hospital Ethnography: Introduction," *Social Science and Medicine* 59 (2004): 1995–2001.

4. See Table 1.2 in Chapter 1, pp. 23-4.

5. To be noted here, though, is the increasing awareness of the complexity of prehistorical cultures and the healing activities of their various specialists—shamans, priests, sorcerers, and herbalists. With this has come the recognition of the significant variety of healing rituals within individual groups and the even more marked variations as one moves across regions and from hunter-gatherer tribes to horticultural and agricultural village societies. These accounts supplement earlier ones that identified shamans as the only healers within "primitive cultures."

    A good beginning point for investigating this matter is the set of six articles on shamanism in *The Encyclopedia of Religion*, 2nd ed., 15 vols., ed. Lindsay Jones (Detroit: Macmillan Reference USA, 2005), vol. 12, pp. 8269–94.

6. We provide a fuller discussion of the "healing response" and the "placebo effect" in Chapter 6.

Chapter 4

1. We have looked to ethnography for guidance in approaching the often-contested territory of religion and healing. For critical questions here, see Larry R. Churchill, "The Dangers of Looking for the Health Benefits of Religion," *Lancet* 369 (2007): 1509–10.

    For a working distinction between "spirituality" and "religion," see Larry R. Churchill, "Religion, Spirituality, and Genetics: Mapping the Terrain for Research Purposes," *American Journal of Medical Genetics* 151C, no. 1 (2008): 6–12.

    Finally, see Robert Bellah on "civil religion" for a discussion of how words charged with religious meaning in specific traditions can evolve into words used in civic, pluralist settings and yet retain their markedly "religious" significance and power. Robert Bellah, "Civil Religion in America," in *The Robert Bellah Reader*, ed. Robert N. Bellah and Steven M. Tipton (Durham, NC: Duke University Press, 2006), pp. 225–45.

2. James Hillman gives this succinct formulation: "the archetypal figure of the Wounded Healer, another ancient and psychological way of expressing that the illness and its healing are one and the same." James Hillman, *Re-Visioning Psychology* (New York: Harper & Row, 1976), p. 76. There is also this profound elaboration in another essay:

> The *wounded healer* does not merely mean that a person has been hurt and can empathize, which is too obvious and never enough to heal. Nor does it mean that a person can heal because he or she has been through an identical process, for this would not help unless the process had utterly altered consciousness. Let us remember that the *wounded healer* is not any human person, but a personification presenting a kind of consciousness. This kind of consciousness refers to mutilations and afflictions of the body organs that release the sparks of consciousness in these organs, resulting in an *organ- or body-consciousness*. Healing comes then not because one is whole, integrated, and all together, but from a consciousness breaking through dismemberment.

James Hillman, "Puer Wounds and Ulysses' Scar," in *Senex and Puer*, ed. Glenn Slater (Dallas, TX: Spring Publications, 2005), p. 234; italics in the original. The entire text of this exceptional essay is much to the point here; pp. 214–47.

Chapter 5

The subtitle to this chapter is taken from Mary O'Flaherty Horn's grim narrative, "On Being a Patient: The Other Side of the Bed Rail," *Annals of Internal Medicine* 130, no. 11 (1999): 940–41. The epigraph comes from Virginia Woolf, *On Being Ill* (Ashfield, MA: Paris Press, 2002), p. 12.

1. Before going further we need to introduce a distinction between illness and disease. Several have made significant contributions to this discussion, but no clinician has written more persuasively about it than Eric Cassell. In his 1976 book *The Healer's Art*, Cassell devotes a chapter to the importance of recognizing that while organs have diseases, it is people who have illnesses. Clinicians, then, should always be about the work of treating people, focusing on their illness even while addressing "the disease." Among contemporary accounts, those of Arthur Frank articulating the patient experience of illness stand out. Illness here is a process of living

in and through and with a body that is behaving in a new way, a strange way—often a distressing and painful way. Diseases, in turn, are terms used within a medical system to point to what is happening in the bodies of patients. See Arthur W. Frank, *At the Will of the Body: Reflections on Illness* (Boston: Houghton Mifflin, 2002), pp. 11–15, et passim. This book is a classic, and deservedly so. We rely on it heavily in this chapter.

Diagnosing disease means accurately naming a bodily state within a medical system. Allopathic medicine operates with one such set of such names, or diagnoses, traditional Chinese medicine with another. Arthur Kleinman's fieldwork in Taiwan and the analytical structure he developed around it are essential for the study of these differences between healthcare systems and for the study of experiences of patients within such systems. See his foundational *Patients and Healers in the Context of Culture: An Exploration of the Borderland between Anthropology, Medicine, and Psychiatry* (Berkeley: University of California Press, 1980).

2. Kleinman, *Patients and Healers*, is especially helpful here. See Chapter 2, pp. 24–70, esp. pp. 49–60.

3. Frank, *At the Will of the Body*, p. 13; italics in the original.

4. Ibid., pp. 13–14.

5. Reynolds Price, *A Whole New Life: An Illness and a Healing* (New York: Atheneum, 1994), pp. 145–46.

6. Ibid., p. 146; italics in the original.

7. Anatole Broyard, *Intoxicated by My Illness: And Other Writings on Life and Death*, comp. and ed. Alexandra Broyard (New York: Clarkson Potter, 1992), p. 40; italics in the original. Broyard's chapter is entitled "The Patient Examines the Doctor."

8. Jill Bolte Taylor, *My Stroke of Insight: A Brain Scientist's Personal Journey* (New York: Viking, 2008), pp. 181–83. For a more complete treatment of all 40 items on the list, see Chapter 13, "What I Needed the Most," pp. 110–21.

9. Children and teenagers, ever so astute, are on to the "naming game." See Michael Nutkiewicz, "Diagnosis versus Dialogue: Oral Testimony and the Study of Pediatric Pain," *Oral History Review* 35, no. 1 (2008)): 11–21. The mean age of the patients in the study was 14. Note the following from p. 17: "I've been told I have a lot of different things. It's funny because each doctor describes it and names it according to his specialty. So if you take the gist of what they're saying, then it's all exactly the same thing . . . "

10. Tessa Willoughby Carr, "Recovering Women: Autobiographical Performances of Illness Experience" (Ph.D. diss., University of Texas at Austin, 2007), p. 186.

11. Price, *Whole New Life*, p. 20.

12. Carr, "Recovering Women," p. 197.

13. Taylor, *My Stroke of Insight*, p. 62.

14. Oliver Sacks, *A Leg to Stand On* (New York: Summit Books, 1984), p. 191; italics in the original. It did not hurt, one imagines, that this physician turned out to have read some of Sacks's books. But, as Sacks makes vividly clear, his standing and reputation did little enough for him in his dealings with his surgeons, attending physicians, and a host of aides, therapists, and nurses.

15. Taylor, *My Stroke of Insight*, p. 84. Again, it probably did not hurt that Dr. Young knew Taylor professionally.

16. Frank, *At the Will of the Body*, p. 26.

17. Susan Miller, "My Left Breast," in *"O Solo Homo": The New Queer Performance*, ed. Holly Hughes and David Román (New York: Grove Press, 1998), pp. 93–120; the quotation is from p. 119.

18. Mark Smith-Soto, *Waiting Room* (Birmingham, AL: Red Mountain Review, 2008), p. 5.

19. Frank, *At the Will of the Body*, pp. 152–53.

20. Broyard, *Intoxicated by My Illness*, p. 56.

21. Ibid., pp. 56–57; italics in the original.

22. Linda Park-Fuller, "A Clean Breast of It," in *Voices Made Flesh: Performing Women's Autobiography*, ed. Lynn C. Miller, Jacqueline Taylor, and M. Heather Carver (Madison: University of Wisconsin Press, 2003), pp. 215–36; the quotation is from p. 225.

23. Kay Redfield Jamison, *An Unquiet Mind: A Memoir of Moods and Madness* (New York: Vintage, 1996), pp. 190–1.

24. Price, *Whole New Life*, p. 13.

25. Taylor, *My Stroke of Insight*, p. 81.

26. Ibid., p. 83.

27. Miller, "My Left Breast," pp. 102–3.

28. Carr, "Recovering Women," pp. 182–95, for this whole account. In the pages that follow, we provide citations only for direct and isolated quotations.

29. Ibid., p. 194.

30. Ibid., pp. 188–92.

31. Ibid., pp. 189–90.

32. Ibid., p. 194.

33. Frank, *At the Will of the Body*, pp. 23–6.

34. For obvious reasons, there is little found in these accounts on bad long-term relationships. But sometimes a person is stuck with a practitioner who simply must be involved. Price and his radiologist are a classic case. See Price, *Whole New Life*, pp. 40–1, 56, 143–4.

35. Norman Cousins, *Anatomy of an Illness as Perceived by the Patient* (New York: W. W. Norton, 1979), p. 49.

36. Ibid., pp. 29–54.

37. Jamison, *Unquiet Mind*, p. 118; first italics in the original, second italics added.

38. Ibid.

39. Price, *Whole New Life*, p. 27.

40. Ibid., pp. 142–3.

41. Nancy Mairs, "On Being a Cripple," in *The Social Medicine Reader*, vol. 2: *Social and Cultural Contributions to Health, Difference, and Inequality*, 2nd ed., ed. Gail E. Henderson, Sue E. Estroff, Larry R. Churchill, Nancy M. P. King, Jonathan Oberlander, and Ronald P. Strauss (Durham, NC: Duke University Press, 2005), pp. 70–81. The following exquisite passage is from pp. 80–1: "Too few doctors, it is true, treat their patients as whole human beings, but the reverse is also true. I have always tried to be gentle with my doctors, who often have more at stake in terms of ego than I do. I may be frustrated, maddened, depressed by the incurability of my disease, but I am not diminished by it, and they are. When I push myself up from my seat in the waiting room and stumble toward them, I incarnate the limitation of their powers. The least I can do is refuse to press on their tenderest spots."

42. Harold Brodkey's marvelous account is *This Wild Darkness: The Story of My Death* (New York: Holt, 1996). We have used passages found throughout the text. Most of the material for this next section is found on pp. 71–91.

43. Ibid., p. 85.

44. Ibid., p. 153.

45. Ibid., p. 177.

46. Frank, *At the Will of the Body*, p. 148; italics added.

47. Taylor, *My Stroke of Insight*, pp. 86–7, et passim.

48. Mairs, "On Being a Cripple," p. 76.

49. Audre Lorde, *The Cancer Journals*, special ed. (San Francisco: Aunt Lute Books, 1997), p. 38.

50. Ibid., p. 29; italics added.

51. Ibid., p. 39.

52. Mairs, "On Being a Cripple," p. 81.

53. Broyard, *Intoxicated by My Illness*, p. 7.

54. Frank, *At the Will of the Body*, p. 120.

55. Lorde, *Cancer Journals*, p. 79.

56. Taylor, *My Stroke of Insight*, p. 82.

57. Frank, *At the Will of the Body*, p. 14.

58. Ibid., p. 54.

59. This is derived from May Sarton's famous remark, "One must think like a hero to behave like a merely decent human being." And then see David Hilfiker, *Not All of Us Are Saints: A Doctor's Journey with the Poor* (New York: Ballantine Books, 1996).

Chapter 6

The epigraph to this chapter comes from Jill Bolte Taylor, *My Stroke of Insight: A Brain Scientist's Personal Journey* (New York: Viking, 2008); italics in the original.

1. Luana Colloca, Leonardo Lopiano, Michele Lanotte, and Fabrizio Benedetti, "Overt versus Covert Treatment for Pain, Anxiety, and Parkinson's Disease," *Lancet Neurology* 3, no. 11 (2004): 679–84.

2. Ted J. Kaptchuk, John M. Kelley, Lisa A. Conboy, Roger B. Davis, Catherine E. Kerr, Eric E. Jacobson, Irving Kirsch, et al., "Components of Placebo Effect: Randomised Controlled Trial in Patients with Irritable Bowel Syndrome," *BMJ* 336 (2008): 999–1003.

3. See Janice K. Kiecolt-Glaser, Lynanne McGuire, Theodore F. Robles, and Ronald Glaser, "Psychoneuroimmunology and Psychosomatic Medicine: Back to the Future," *Psychosomatic Medicine* 64 (2002): 15–28; and J. K. Kiecolt-Glaser, T. F. Robles, K. L. Heffner, T. J. Loving, and R. Glaser, "Psycho-oncology and Cancer: Psychoneuroimmunology and Cancer," *Annals of Oncology* 13, suppl. 4 (2002): 165–9.

4. Eve Henry, "The Healing Response and the Doctor-Patient Relationship: Enhancing Treatment through Alterations of Contextual Factors" (unpublished paper, Vanderbilt University, 2008).

5. Fabrizio Benedetti, Antonella Pollo, Leonardo Lopiano, Michele Lanotte, Sergio Vighetti, and Innocenzo Rainero, "Conscious Expectation and Unconscious Conditioning in Analgesic, Motor, and Hormonal Placebo/ Nocebo Responses," *Journal of Neuroscience* 23, no. 10 (2003): 4315–23.

6. Ibrahim Hashish, Ho Kee Hai, Wilson Harvey, Charlotte Feinmann, and Malcolm Harris, "Reduction of Postoperative Pain and Swelling by Ultrasound Treatment: A Placebo Effect," *Pain* 33, no. 3 (1988): 303–11.

7. D. P. Phillips, T. E. Ruth, and L. M. Wagner, "Psychology and Survival," *Lancet* 342 (1993): 1142–5.

8. See Nicholas J. Voudouris, Connie L. Peck, and Grahame Coleman, "Conditioned Response Models of Placebo Phenomena: Further Support," *Pain* 38, no. 1 (1989): 109–16, and Nicholas J. Voudouris, Connie L. Peck, and Grahame Coleman, "The Role of Conditioning and Verbal Expectancy in the Placebo Response," *Pain* 43, no. 1 (1990): 121–8.

9. Donald D. Price, "Placebo Analgesia," in *Psychological Mechanisms of Pain and Analgesia* (Seattle: IASP Press, 1999), pp. 155–82.

10. Earl K. Miller and Jonathan D. Cohen, "An Integrative Theory of Prefrontal Cortex Function," *Annual Review of Neuroscience* 24 (2001): 167–202.

11. Jon-Kar Zubieta, Joshua A. Bueller, Lisa R. Jackson, David J. Scott, Yanjun Xu, Robert A. Koeppe, Thomas E. Nichols, and Christian S. Stohler, "Placebo Effects Mediated by Endogenous Opioid Activity on μ-Opioid Receptors," *Journal of Neuroscience* 25, no. 34 (2005): 7754–62.

12. Predrag Petrovic and Martin Ingvar, "Imaging Cognitive Modulation of Pain Processing," *Pain* 95, nos. 1–2 (2002): 1–5.

13. Tor D. Wager, James K. Rilling, Edward E. Smith, Alex Sokolik, Kenneth L. Casey, Richard J. Davidson, Stephen M. Kosslyn, Robert M. Rose, and Jonathan D. Cohen, "Placebo-Induced Changes in fMRI in the Anticipation and Experience of Pain," *Science* 303 (2004): 1162–7.

14. Predrag Petrovic, Thomas Dietrich, Peter Fransson, Jesper Andersson, Katrina Carlsson, and Martin Ingvar, "Placebo in Emotional Processing— Induced Expectations of Anxiety Relief Activate a Generalized Modulatory Network," *Neuron* 46 (2005): 957–69.

15. See Wager et al., "Placebo-Induced Changes in fMRI."

16. See ibid.

17. Jack B. Nitschke, Gregory E. Dixon, Issidoros Sarinopoulos, Sarah J. Short, Jonathan D. Cohen, Edward E. Smith, Stephen M. Kosslyn, Robert M. Rose, and Richard J. Davidson, "Altering Expectancy Dampens Neural Response to Aversive Taste in Primary Taste Cortex," *Nature Neuroscience* 9, no. 3 (2006): 435–42.

18. Ronald Melzack and Patrick D. Wall, "Pain Mechanisms: A New Theory," *Science* 150 (1965): 971–9.

19. See Petrovic and Ingvar, "Imaging Cognitive Modulation of Pain Processing"; Petrovic et al., "Placebo in Emotional Processing"; and Wager et al., "Placebo-Induced Changes in fMRI."

20. Eric R. Kandel, James H. Schwartz, and Thomas M. Jessell, *Principles of Neural Science*, 4th ed. (New York: McGraw-Hill, Health Professions Division, 2000).

21. Franklin G. Miller and Ted J. Kaptchuk, "The Power of Context: Reconceptualizing the Placebo Effect," *Journal of the Royal Society of Medicine* 101 (2008): 222–25.

22. Anthropologist Daniel Moerman also argues this point and makes a case for the term "meaning response" as a more felicitous way to describe this set of phenomena. See Daniel E. Moerman, *Meaning, Medicine, and the "Placebo Effect"* (New York: Cambridge University

Press, 2002). We have learned much from Moerman's work but prefer the term "healing response," as we will argue later in this chapter.

23. Miller and Kaptchuk, "Power of Context." See also the important work of Howard Brody on placebos and the placebo effect over the past several decades, including *Placebos and the Philosophy of Medicine: Clinical, Conceptual, and Ethical Issues* (Chicago: University of Chicago Press, 1980); "The Placebo Response. Part I: Exploring the Myths; Part II: Use in Clinical Practice," *Drug Therapy* 16, no. 7 (1986): 106–31; and "The Doctor as Therapeutic Agent: A Placebo Effect Research Agenda," in *The Placebo Effect: An Interdisciplinary Exploration*, ed. Anne Harrington (Cambridge, MA: Harvard University Press, 1997), 77–92. In this last essay Brody draws a conclusion still couched in the idiom of placebos but compatible with our thesis in this book: "We should employ the psychological and social sciences to determine which circumstances of human social interaction alter the meaning of an illness experience for a given patient in a possible direction, thus setting a placebo response in motion" (87).

24. Richard J. Davidson, "Well-Being and Affective Style: Neural Substrates and Biobehavioural Correlates," *Philosophical Transactions of the Royal Society of London*, ser. B, 359 (2004): 1395–411.

25. Richard J. Davidson, Jon Kabat-Zinn, Jessica Schumacher, Melissa Rosenkranz, Daniel Muller, Saki F. Santorelli, Ferris Urbanowski, Anne Harrington, Katherine Bonus, and John F. Sheridan, "Alterations in Brain and Immune Function Produced by Mindfulness Meditation," *Psychosomatic Medicine* 65 (2003): 564–70.

26. Edward J. Huth and T. Jock Murray, *Medicine in Quotations: Views of Health and Disease through the Ages*, 2nd ed. (Philadelphia: American College of Physicians, 2006).

27. Michael W. Rabow, Rachel N. Remen, Dean X. Parmelee, and Thomas S. Inui, "Professional Formation: Extending Medicine's Lineage of Service into the Next Century," *Academic Medicine* 85, no. 2 (2010): 310–7.

28. Carol P. Tresolini and the Pew-Fetzer Task Force, *Health Professions Education and Relationship-Centered Care* (San Francisco: Pew Health Professions Commission, 1994).

29. Institute of Medicine Committee on Quality Health Care in America, *Crossing the Quality Chasm: A New Health System for the 21st Century* (Washington, DC: National Academy Press, 2001).

30. See, for example, R. C. Smith, A. M. Dorsey, J. S. Lyles, and R. M. Frankel, "Teaching Self-Awareness Enhances Learning about Patient-Centered Interviewing," *Academic Medicine* 74, no. 11 (1999): 1242–8, and S. Williams, J. Weinman, and J. Dale, "Doctor-Patient

Communication and Patient Satisfaction: A Review," *Family Practice* 15 (1998): 480–92.

31. D. H. Novack, R. M. Epstein, and R. H. Paulsen, "Toward Creating Physician-Healers: Fostering Medical Students' Self-Awareness, Personal Growth, and Well-Being," *Academic Medicine* 74, no. 5 (1999): 516–20.

32. Daniel J. Siegel, *The Mindful Brain: Reflection and Attunement in the Cultivation of Well-Being* (New York: W. W. Norton, 2007), p. 17.

33. Sharon Dobie, "Viewpoint: Reflections on a Well-Traveled Path: Self-Awareness, Mindful Practice, and Relationship-Centered Care as Foundations for Medical Education," *Academic Medicine* 82, no. 4 (2007): 422–27.

Chapter 7

The epigraph to this chapter comes from Jon Kabat-Zinn, foreword to *Heal Thy Self: Lessons on Mindfulness in Medicine*, by Saki Santorelli (New York: Bell Tower, 1999), p. xxiv.

1. Anatole Broyard, *Intoxicated by My Illness: And Other Writings on Life and Death*, comp. and ed. Alexandra Broyard (New York: Clarkson Potter, 1992), pp. 33–58.

2. Jodi Halpern, *From Detached Concern to Empathy: Humanizing Medical Practice* (New York: Oxford University Press, 2001), p. 60.

3. Debra L. Roter, Moira Stewart, Samuel M. Putnam, Mack Lipkin Jr., William Stiles, and Thomas S. Inui, "Communication Patterns of Primary Care Physicians," *Journal of the American Medical Association* 277 (1997): 350–6.

4. Halpern, *From Detached Concern to Empathy*, pp. 80ff.

5. Ibid., p. 93.

6. Ibid., p. 94.

7. Broyard, *Intoxicated by My Illness*, p. 57.

8. Ibid.

Chapter 8

The epigraphs to this chapter come from César Vallejo, *The Black Heralds*, trans. Rebecca Seiferle (Port Townsend, WA: Copper Canyon Press, 2003), p. 3; Cicero, quoted in Pierre Hadot, *Philosophy as a Way of Life: Spiritual Exercises from Socrates to Foucault*, ed. Arnold I. Davidson, trans.

Michael Chase (Oxford: Blackwell, 1995), p. 110, n. 15; and *The Art and Thought of Heraclitus: An Edition of the Fragments with Translation and Commentary*, ed. Charles H. Kahn (Cambridge: Cambridge University Press, 1979), p. 81 (more exactly, from p. 260: *ēthos anthrōpōi daimōn*—"character, for man [is his] *daimōn*").

1. For amplification see Larry R. Churchill, Nancy M. P. King, and David Schenck, "Ethics in Medicine: An Introduction to Moral Tools and Traditions," in *The Social Medicine Reader*, vol. 1: *Patients, Doctors, and Illness*, 2nd ed., ed. Nancy M. P. King, Ronald P. Strauss, Larry R. Churchill, Sue E. Estroff, Gail E. Henderson, and Jonathan Oberlander (Durham, NC: Duke University Press, 2005), pp. 169–85.

2. Michael Polanyi, *Personal Knowledge: Towards a Post-Critical Philosophy* (New York: Harper & Row, 1964), pp. 54–55.

3. Hadot, *Philosophy as a Way of Life*, p. 83; italics in the original.

4. Ibid., pp. 82–3. See also pp. 81–2 for Hadot's helpful elucidation of puzzles of usage and translation lying behind his choice of the phrase "spiritual exercises."

5. Ibid., p. 31.

6. To be sure, the advent of bioethics in the 1960s ushered in a new period of practical relevance for philosophy, or more precisely ethical philosophy, in the form of renewed interest in the practical moral problems of medicine and the life sciences. Variously termed "medical ethics," "bioethics," or "responsible conduct of research," this late-20th-century and early-21st-century enterprise has, in the words of Stephen Toulmin, "saved the life of ethics" by returning it to its role as a set of tools of immediate relevance to some of the knottiest problems we face. See his "How Medicine Saved the Life of Ethics," in *Perspectives in Biology and Medicine* 25, no. 4 (1982): 736-50. Among these are the uses of an increasingly robust technology for intervening and changing human life from prenatal existence to the deathbed, and beyond. Yet the new relevance for ethics in medicine, medical science, and research has not moved far beyond pronouncements on this well-rehearsed set of issues spawned by more powerful technologies. The new practical ethics in medicine and science, while clearly an advance in relevance, seems to have been purchased at the price of confining ethics to the conceptual analysis of dilemmas. No one has been clearer about this than Edmund Pincoffs in his disparaging characterization of modern ethics as "quandary ethics."

> Quandary ethics is a newcomer. . . . the 'quandarist' is fighting a very long tradition with which he is at odds. Plato, Aristotle, the Epicureans,

> the Stoics, Augustine, Aquinas, Shaftesbury, Hume and Hegel do not
> conceive of ethics as quandarists do.

Note how encompassing this list is that Pincoffs offers—ancient, medieval, and modern.

> If they [the philosophers listed] are read for their theories—that is, for the grounds that they give for making particularly difficult moral decisions—their teachings are inevitably distorted. To give such grounds, such justifications of particular difficult decisions, was not their objective. They were ... concerned with moral enlightenment, education and the good for man.

> Edmund L. Pincoffs, *Quandaries and Virtues: Against Reductivism in Ethics* (Lawrence: University Press of Kansas, 1986), pp. 14–5.

> For our purposes the critical point is this: Though in contemporary discussion the understanding of philosophy as a way of life is far from being the dominant model, over the historical span of Western philosophy this understanding can be seen to be the dominant theme and practice.

> While it would be wrong to gainsay the contributions that have been made by the modern enterprise of bioethics, gone from the professional and popular imagination is the idea of ethics as something not only practical but much deeper than a set of problem-solving tools.

7. Our account is drawn primarily from Hadot's critical chapter, "Spiritual Exercises," in *Philosophy as a Way of Life*, pp. 81–125. For our purposes, other key Hadot texts include "Forms of Life and Forms of Discourse in Ancient Philosophy," in ibid., pp. 49–70, and "The *Meditations* as Spiritual Exercises," in Pierre Hadot, *The Inner Citadel: The "Meditations" of Marcus Aurelius*, trans. Michael Chase (Cambridge, MA: Harvard University Press, 1998), pp. 35–53. In addition see Pierre Hadot, *What Is Ancient Philosophy?*, trans. Michael Chase (Cambridge, MA: Harvard University Press, 2002).

8. Hadot also describes preparatory exercises of Epicureans, including the memorization of maxims; the study of Epicurean physics; the turning of the mind from unpleasant things to pleasurable ones, from bad memories to good; and friendship itself. *Philosophy as a Way of Life*, pp. 87–9.

9. Ibid., p. 85; translator's insertion. Note below Hadot's reservations about his use of the term "meditation," which should be read alongside his hesitation about the use of "spiritual exercises" referenced above in note 4. Both are examples of the terminological and conceptual

difficulties entailed in explicating this interpretation of ancient philosophy, given contemporary usages:

> It is only after much hesitation that I have translated *melete* by "meditation." In fact *melete* and its Latin equivalent *meditatio* designate "preparatory exercises." . . . We must not, however, lose sight of the term's ambiguity: meditation is exercise, and exercise is meditation.

Hadot, *Philosophy as a Way of Life*, p. 112, n. 38; italics in the original. We will on occasion, as in the passage just quoted in our text, take the liberty of substituting "preparatory exercises" for "meditation."

10. Hadot, *Philosophy as a Way of Life*, p. 85.
11. Ibid.
12. Ibid., p. 86. For elaboration of this matter of the everydayness of ethics and related points in our discussion of Hadot from a completely different disciplinary perspective, see cognitive scientist Francisco J. Varela's *Ethical Know-How: Action, Wisdom, and Cognition* (Stanford, CA: Stanford University Press, 1999). On the "everydayness of ethics" in particular, see pp. 4–6, and then the entire second lecture, "On Ethical Expertise," pp. 23–41. Useful background for *Ethical Know-How*, which is a very tightly argued, rapidly moving text of 85 pages, may be found in Francisco J. Varela, Evan Thompson, and Eleanor Rosch, *The Embodied Mind: Cognitive Science and Human Experience* (Cambridge, MA: MIT Press, 1993).
13. Hadot, *Philosophy as a Way of Life*, p. 102.
14. Ibid., pp. 104–6. Again, compare Varela's discussion in *Ethical Know-How*, "Lessons from the Teaching Traditions," pp. 65–75, which can easily be read as a commentary on and further development of Hadot's depiction of the teaching traditions of Hellenistic and Roman philosophy. For instance:

> How can such an attitude of all-encompassing, de-centered, responsive, compassionate concern be fostered and embodied in our culture? It obviously cannot be created merely through norms and rationalistic injunctions. It must be developed and embodied through *disciplines* that facilitate the letting-go of ego-centered habits and enable compassion to become spontaneous and self-sustaining. (p. 73; italics in the original)

We simply cannot overlook the need for some form of sustained, disciplined practice or *pratique de transformation de sujet*, to use Foucault's apt term. This is not something that one can make up for oneself—anymore than one can make up the history of Western science for oneself. Nothing will take its place. (pp. 74–5)

Of note in our context is Varela's acknowledgment of Michel Foucault's examination of ancient philosophy in *The History of Sexuality*, trans. Robert Hurley, 3 vols. (New York: Vintage, 1988–90). One then finds in Foucault's text favorable mention of Hadot. And Hadot devotes a chapter of *Philosophy as a Way of Life* to analyzing this work of Foucault's: see "Reflections on the Idea of the 'Cultivation of the Self,'" pp. 206–13. We would encourage the reader interested in Foucault's perspective on ancient philosophy as a matter of practice and self-formation also to consult Michel Foucault, *The Hermeneutics of the Subject: Lectures at the Collège de France, 1981–1982*, ed. Frédéric Gros, trans. Graham Burchell (New York: Picador, 2005); see esp. lectures 13 (pp. 247–69), 15 (pp. 289–314), and 18 (pp. 355–70).

15. Hadot, *Philosophy as a Way of Life*, p. 83.
16. All four quotations are from ibid.: Epicurus, p. 87; Cicero, Epicurus, and Epictetus, p. 110, n. 15.
17. See Jonathan Imber's perspicacious account of the fortunes of character in the development of allopathic medicine in the United States. Jonathan B. Imber, *Trusting Doctors: The Decline of Moral Authority in American Medicine* (Princeton, NJ: Princeton University Press, 2008).
18. With the introduction of "character traits" as natural correlations with healing skills, some readers may begin to think in terms of virtues and virtue theory. A well-known and helpful work on the virtues of practitioners is Edmund Pellegrino and David Thomasma's *The Virtues in Medical Practice* (New York: Oxford University Press, 1993), which enumerates and argues for a set of virtues they believe are central to the activity of doctoring. We have chosen to avoid framing our findings within the interpretative scheme of virtues, since that would take us in a more theoretical direction, one familiar in bioethics, in which the major concern is to justify a virtue-oriented approach in contrast to a principlist orientation to medical ethics. Our approach in this volume is empirical and interpretative, rather than theoretical. Our focus is on what clinicians have said, rather than on which list of virtues can be defended on Aristotelian, Thomistic, or other grounds.

INDEX